DENTAL SCIENCE, MATERIALS AND TECHNOLOGY

ORAL HEALTH

ANESTHETIC MANAGEMENT, SOCIAL DETERMINANTS, ROLE OF NUTRITION AND IMPACT ON QUALITY OF LIFE

DENTAL SCIENCE, MATERIALS AND TECHNOLOGY

Additional books in this series can be found on Nova's website under the Series tab.

Additional e-books in this series can be found on Nova's website under the e-book tab.

DENTAL SCIENCE, MATERIALS AND TECHNOLOGY

ORAL HEALTH

ANESTHETIC MANAGEMENT, SOCIAL DETERMINANTS, ROLE OF NUTRITION AND IMPACT ON QUALITY OF LIFE

JULIA RENEE BARNES
EDITOR

NOVA BIOMEDICAL

New York

Library of Congress Cataloging-in-Publication Data

ISBN: 978-1-63482-832-1
Library of Congress Control Number: 2015939091

Published by Nova Science Publishers, Inc. † New York

Contents

Preface

Biological, psychological, sociological and ecological features of life contribute and interact simultaneously in the development of an individual's oral health. The chapters in this book review the effects of periodontal disease and its treatment on OHRQoL (Oral Health-Related Quality of Life); the consequences of periodontal disease and patient perceptions of the impact of their gingival/periodontal health on their everyday lives; the link between nutritional factors and periodontal disease; a review of Charcot-Marie-Tooth Disease (CMTD), the most common sensitive and motor peripheral neuropathy; the influence of improved oral health literacy considering the circumstances in which a person has been born, lives and works, the microbiological mechanisms, and the public's influence to improve oral health; the complexities related to oral care of people who experience mental disorders and the implications this may hold for their quality of life, practice, research and policy; determinants of oral health in schizophrenic patients; and an assessment of the PIDAQ (Psychosocial Impact of Dental Aesthetic Questionnaire), the only available tool designed specifically to assess malocclusions.

Chapter I – Periodontal disease is an inflammatory disease initiated by mixed opportunistic bacterial pathogens in the dental plaque biofilm. In the susceptible patient, advancing periodontal disease often leads to loss of supporting soft and hard tissues around a tooth. Due to the nature and progression of the disease, methods of characterizing periodontal disease have often been based on clinical parameters such as probing pockets depths, clinical attachment levels, bleeding on probing, mobility scores and gingival recession. Unfortunately, such parameters show no indication of how the disease affects the patients themselves. Of recent years, patient centered assessments such as Oral Health-Related Quality of Life (OHRQoL) are increasingly appreciated and being applied. Such measures incorporate the functional, psychological and social consequences of oral conditions for the individual, and not merely signs and symptoms of the disease itself. This chapter will review the effects of periodontal disease and its treatment on OHRQoL. Patients often report functional limitation, physical pain and psychological disability associated with the signs and symptoms of periodontal disease. Such effects on OHRQoL have been shown to diminish with proper treatment. Furthermore, recent studies have also shown that the complications or outcome of different treatment strategies have, to varying degrees, an effect on patients daily life. These complications such as tooth loss, recession and pain are closely related and interplay to affect the patient's OHRQoL.

Chapter II – Periodontal diseases are one of the common oral diseases involving structural and functional changes in the oral cavity and in their most severe forms are associated with formation of periodontal pockets, gingival abscesses, gingival recessions, tooth mobility, and finally teeth loss. Periodontal diseases are one of the main reasons for tooth loss among the population and this is furthermore related not only to alteration in speaking and chewing functions, but also to a high impact on the patients psychological and emotional well-being as related to daily social interactions, organ loss related trauma, self-esteem, shame, depression, anxiety. As a consequence, a better understanding of the consequences of periodontal disease is important in understanding patient perceptions of the impact of their gingival/periodontal health on their everyday lives, in planning periodontal therapy which addresses patient needs and in evaluating the results of the periodontal treatment from the patient's perspective. In the last decades, the relationship between individuals' periodontal health/therapy and quality of life has been extensively examined and this chapter reviews the current knowledge in this research field.

Chapter III – Periodontal diseases are one of the common oral diseases and it is associated with formation of periodontal pockets, gingival abscesses, gingival recessions, tooth mobility, and finally teeth loss. The link between nutritional factors and periodontal disease has not been clearly established even if a highly number of studies has investigated this possible association. As periodontitis is associated with low serum/plasma micronutrient levels, it has been postulated that daily intake for vitamin C (ascorbic acid), vitamin E, zinc, lycopene, vitamin B, complex vitamin D, calcium, unsaturated fats and antioxidants would have useful adjunct benefits on the prevention and therapeutic management of periodontal disease. Regarding various beverages, the consumption of milk, coffee or green tea was also investigated in relationship with periodontitis. It has been showed that higher coffee consumption is associated with a significant reduction in number of teeth with periodontal bone loss, while green tea extract has been revealed to suppress the onset of loss of attachment and alveolar bone resorption in a rat model of experimental periodontitis. This chapter reviews the current knowledge in this research field, suggesting an adequate dietary advice for patients with chronic periodontitis.

Chapter IV – Biological, psychological, sociological, and ecological features of life contribute and interact simultaneously in the development of an individual's oral health. For example, a person's oral health is influenced by culture/race/ethnicity, neighborhood/rural area, government structure (with programs for education and healthcare), and level of social cohesion/power (support from friends, family, church members, community members, etc.), all of which may vary over the person's life, *as well as* brushing and flossing, proper nutrition, immunological status, saliva production, oral microbes, etc. When group variations in preventable disease differ primarily due to social conditions, the situation is described as a health disparity due to the social determinants of health. In the U.S., public policymakers are expected to address such group health differences through: the promotion of education; safe/healthy homes, schools, and workplaces; reduction of poverty; and the reduction of discrimination (racial-based, gender-based, age-based, etc.) in addition to: the encouragement of life-style changes to lessen risk; healthcare; and research. The purpose of this chapter is to review the influence of improved oral health literacy considering the circumstances in which a person has been born, lives, and works (social determinants), the microbiological mechanisms, and the public's influence to improve oral health.

Chapter V – Mental disorders represent one of the largest burdens of disease globally. People who experience mental illness have incrementally worse physical health compared to the general population. While there is a movement in mental health care to consider physical health needs of service users, the oral health needs are not routinely assessed. Compounding the lack of routine or standardised oral health assessment in mental health services, service users/consumers often demonstrate avoidant health seeking behaviours. Health service avoidance for physical care needs is often compounded by prohibitive costs, stigma related to mental disorder, unsatisfactory previous encounters with oral care practitioners and psychiatric symptomatology impacting behaviours. This chapter will using contemporary literature describe the complexities related to oral care of people who experience mental disorders and the implications this may hold for their quality of life, practice, research and policy.

Chapter VI – Schizophrenia is a severe mental disorder. It is a ubiquitous disease affecting 1% of the world population. Delusions and hallucinations are symptoms of the disease, but discordance and negation of the body mean these people are not always able to make the right decisions to take care of their health. This is one reason why dental health indicators are very high compared to the general population. Poor oral health is one of the causes of stigma from which these people suffer greatly. Determinants of the oral health of these patients are multiple. The neurological effects of first-generation antipsychotic drugs are multiple (dyskinesia, extrapyramidal syndrome, myasthenia gravis, and trismus) and disrupt the motricity of the oral region. The metabolic effects of second-generation antipsychotic drugs (dyslipidemia, hyperglycemia, weight gain, hyperprolactinemia, and cardiovascular ischemic disorders) and more generally anti-cholinergic pharmacopoeia worsen dental problems further. There are also other determinants of oral health of schizophrenic patients, such as disruption of the nociceptive pathways, taking psychoactive substances, smoking, poor diet and lifestyle, and lower socioeconomic status. The lack of somatic care in relation to the division between body and mind must also be mentioned. Lastly, health promotion activities are inadequate for these populations and health professionals lack training in this area. Studies on the subject are difficult to implement because patients do not readily consent to the exploration of an organ with a strong symbolic and emotional component. Studies that target only schizophrenic patients are few and far between and only concern hospitalized patients, i.e. few patients. The state of knowledge in this area has a low level of evidence. Outstanding issues are numerous regarding the effectiveness of preventive actions and management of patients with very specific needs. In this context, we analyzed the impact of poor oral health of schizophrenic patients on their overall health and quality of life through motivational and cognitive constraints imposed by the symptoms of schizophrenia, but also through the unique perspective of caregivers and society about this disease that is too often stigmatized.

Chapter VII – Objectives: *Psychosocial Impact of Dental Aesthetic Questionnaire* (PIDAQ) represents the only available tool for assessing the quality of life for the orthodontic patients. The research studied the relationships between the different aspects of orthodontic care planning, and validated the Romanian version of the PIDAQ questionnaire. Material and methods: A transversal study was carried out on a sample of 1126 subjects, age ranging between 6 and 28 years old. The self-evaluation of the orthodontic esthetic perception was assessed with the PIDAQ index, and the orthodontic treatment need was measured with the IOTN index. Results: Esthetic perception - 70% of the subjects are unsatisfied with the appearance of their dentition. Orthodontic treatment need perception - All the subjects consider that they need orthodontic treatment. Esthetic perception and orthodontic treatment need relationship - 40.16% of the subjects, which were unsatisfied with their dentition appearance, considered that they do not require an orthodontic treatment. Esthetic perception and the esthetic component of IOTN correlation - Among the subjects, assessed as in need severe treatment, 80% were “Unsatisfied” or ”Deeply unsatisfied” with their dentition. Discussion: The scores of the different PIDAQ dimensions determined in our study, were comparable with those reported by other authors. Conclusion: The PIDAQ questionnaire remains the only tool to assess the link between the dental-maxillary anomalies and the quality of life. Our results demonstrate that the Romanian version of the PIDAQ questionnaire is a valid instrument in assessing the psychosocial impact of the dentition esthetics related to the malocclusion.

In: Oral Health
Editor: Julia Renee Barnes
ISBN: 978-1-63482-832-1

Chapter I

Periodontal Disease and Oral Health-Related Quality of Life

Victor Goh[1,2], Dipti Nihalani[1,3] and W. Keung Leung[1]
[1]Faculty of Dentistry, The University of Hong Kong, Hong Kong SAR, China
[2]Faculty of Dentistry, The National University of Malaysia, Malaysia
[3]Zircon Dental Center, Doha, Qatar

Abstract

Periodontal disease is an inflammatory disease initiated by mixed opportunistic bacterial pathogens in the dental plaque biofilm. In the susceptible patient, advancing periodontal disease often leads to loss of supporting soft and hard tissues around a tooth. Due to the nature and progression of the disease, methods of characterizing periodontal disease have often been based on clinical parameters such as probing pockets depths, clinical attachment levels, bleeding on probing, mobility scores and gingival recession. Unfortunately, such parameters show no indication of how the disease affects the patients themselves. Of recent years, patient centered assessments such as Oral Health-Related Quality of Life (OHRQoL) are increasingly appreciated and being applied. Such measures incorporate the functional, psychological and social consequences of oral conditions for the individual, and not merely signs and symptoms of the disease itself. This chapter will review the effects of periodontal disease and its treatment on OHRQoL. Patients often report functional limitation, physical pain and psychological disability associated with the signs and symptoms of periodontal disease. Such effects on OHRQoL have been shown to diminish with proper treatment. Furthermore, recent studies have also shown that the complications or outcome of different treatment strategies have, to varying degrees, an effect on patients daily life. These complications such as tooth loss, recession and pain are closely related and interplay to affect the patient's OHRQoL.

Keywords: Quality of Life, periodontitis

1. Introduction

Oral diseases have significant effects on one's physical and psychological health. The experience of pain or discomfort, difficulty with eating, smiling and other social interactions due to damaged, missing, abnormal or diseased oral structures have profound consequences on people's daily lives and general well-being. Such symptoms restrict activities at work, school or even at home leading to loss of millions of productive hours annually. This is a persistent global problem particularly among underprivileged groups in both developing and developed countries (Reisine, 1984, Gift et al., 1992, Petersen et al., 2005).

The dental literature has in many years been dedicated to constructing and validating sensitive and accurate indices for classifying oral diseases, or rather, the clinical picture of the diseases. Unfortunately, they give us no indication of how these clinician-determined parameters affect the patient's daily lives and nothing about subjectively perceived disease outcomes such as pain, discomfort, psychological and social impacts (Locker, 1988). As such quality of life (QoL) measures have become an important tool to assess a patient's physical, psychological and social well-being (Wilson and Cleary, 1995).

The World Health Organization (WHO) defined QoL as:

> "Individuals' perception of their position in life in the context of the culture and value systems in which they live and in relation to their goals, expectations, standards and concerns"

QoL is a multidimensional concept, incorporating in a complex way ones' physical health, psychological state, level of independence, social relationships, personal beliefs and their relationships to salient features of their environment.

The WHO's definition emphasizes the fact that QoL is a broad-ranged and subjective construct which includes both positive and negative facets of life (WHO, 1995).

As the health profession continues to see an emerging importance in incorporating patient's QoL in treatment planning, approval of new therapies and policy research (WHO, 1995), this chapter will discuss the importance of such measures in the dental field and how these measures are used in understanding the impact of periodontal disease on patient's QoL.

2. Burden of Dental Disease on Society

Periodontal disease and tooth decay have for decades been a huge burden on global oral health. Even today, dental caries is still a major oral health problem as it affects up to 90% of school-aged children and a vast majority of adults worldwide (Petersen et al., 2005, Bagramian et al., 2009). In less developed regions of the world and among the less affluent populations in industrialized countries, both children and adults suffering from severe dental caries are often denied proper treatment. Due to social disparity, financial constraints and inadequacy in available oral health services, decayed teeth are often left untreated or simply extracted to relief pain (Petersen et al., 2005, Bagramian et al., 2009).

Similarly, periodontal disease is considered a major oral health problem with its severe form affecting approximately 11% of the world's population (Richards, 2014) with most children and adolescents worldwide having signs of gingivitis (Petersen et al., 2005). Imagine that 1 out of 10 people may be affected by advance periodontal disease. At an individual level, the burden of periodontal disease on daily function may not be substantial. However, when taken at a population level, the cumulative consequences of the disease may have significant ramifications on social function (Locker, 1988). Given the high prevalence of periodontal diseases, work loss due to the debilitating effects of the disease, and the need for time consuming therapy becomes substantial (Locker and Miller, 1994).

Such effects may be seen in the initial works by Reisine (1984) on dental disease and work loss. She stated that out of 2,600 working adults interviewed, a quarter reported at least one episode of work loss in the previous 12 months related to oral health problems and need for dental treatment visits with an average time lost from work of 1.7 hours (Reisine, 1984). Though a mere 1-2 hours of work loss yearly by a single person may not have severe social implications, when such a measure is calculated at a larger population level, the impact of dental disorders on work loss becomes significant enough to cause certain social and economic dysfunction (Reisine, 1984, Gift et al., 1992)

Gift and co-workers (1992) reported that in 1989, at the national level, an annual work loss of 164 million hours was accumulated by working adults in the United States due to personal oral problems or need for dental visits. In terms of missing school hours, they stated that more than 51 million study hours were lost in a single year by school-age children as a result of oral diseases or dental visits. Among those who missed work or some school time, a similar pattern was observed where females, lower socio-economic classes, and those without health insurance were found to have lost more hours (Gift et al., 1992).

Due to vast disparities in socioeconomic status, the lower income groups have often been denied proper oral health care as a result of financial constraints and lower education levels. These inequalities may lead to differences in perceived needs, and attitudes about oral health (Hosseinpoor et al., 2012, Tchicaya and Lorentz, 2014).

3. Emerging Importance of Patient Centred Outcome Measures

Though the report by Reisine's (1984) group was not restricted to periodontal disease, it does shine a light upon the debilitating effects such diseases have on society. Chronic diseases such as periodontal disease have been shown to exert substantial economic impact on both the health care system and the individual patient (Yach et al., 2004). Vernazza and colleagues (2012) discussed in detail the economics of treating periodontal disease. Economic assessments are concerned with evaluating inputs with outcomes, or costs with benefits (Vernazza et al., 2012). As the complicated scope of health economics is not the topic of discussion here, a simpler way to look at things would be that the more benefits one could gain for a specific cost, the more effective that treatment strategy would be. In line with the World Health Organization's definition of health as being a state of complete physical, mental and social well-being and not merely the absence of disease or infirmity (WHO, 1948), patient-reported outcomes on top of clinical measures are becoming an important focus for researchers and policy makers alike to determine the most effective way of utilizing often scarce resources to gain maximum benefits.

Although periodontal diseases are rarely a matter of life and death, growing indications that oral diseases as such might have significant ramifications on social, psychological and fiscal areas of life are making way for more complicated treatment outcome measures such as impact on QoL to be applied in its therapy. Systematic and quantitative information on the impact of oral disease on QoL would prove useful for several reasons (Nikias, 1985):

I. Such measures would be valuable in making decisions when allocating scarce resources for delivery of health care.
II. For a more comprehensive understanding of oral health problems, a broader range of knowledge regarding the consequences of disease is essential.
III. Patient's perception regarding the social, economic, and psychological consequences of oral diseases may play an important role in changing their oral health practices, including routine and preventive use of dental care.

Indeed what these three points pointed out are important when selecting treatment strategies and educating patients of specific target groups regarding oral health. For instances, Gift and colleagues (1992) stated that perceptions of need for care and the use of home remedies varies between socioeconomic classes. Individuals from lower socioeconomic groups tend to use home remedies or engage in self-care more often to avoid or at least delay the need for professional treatment, while individuals from higher socioeconomic groups engage in self-care to complement professional care (Gift et al., 1992). Such observations highlight the fact that patients from lower socioeconomic backgrounds may seek dental treatment only for curative measures to relief pain as a last resort (Antunes et al., 2003). Due to differences in oral health believes and practices, when providing treatment and educating such patients on the need for periodontal therapy, the use of clinical measures may not matter much. Discussion about probing depths or clinical attachment loss may not be of interest to this patient group, but a risk of pain, disruption in their ability to eat, speak or even work due to disease might prove to be more easily understood and appear more significant in their daily lives. In shorter terms, for any therapy to be considered successful, both the diagnosis and the suggested therapy must make sense in terms of the patient's lay models of illness (Helman, 1981).

When choosing treatment options for lower income groups, the growing evidence on the impact of treatment strategies on patient reported outcome measures may also be applied. For example, Wong et al., (2012) showed that non-surgical periodontal therapy not only was able to improve clinical parameters of moderate-to-advance chronic periodontitis, when patient centred outcomes were evaluated, improvements in terms of patient perceived physical pain, etc. were observed. Mombelli et al., (2011) concluded that use of adjunctive antibiotics can enhance the clinical outcome of non-surgical periodontal treatment, which may reduce the need for surgery. While Flemmig and Beikler (2013) pointed out that the cost of non-surgical periodontal treatment with adjunctive antibiotics is much lower than that of periodontal flap surgery.

Though these treatment modalities may not be equal in efficacy, such emerging evidence can aid clinicians and policy makers in deciding treatment strategies and allocation of resources for lower socioeconomic groups. In this case, since both treatment modalities are clinically effective, and non-surgical periodontal treatment alone is enough to improve patient reported outcomes at a lower cost, clinicians may emphasize on such strategies when treating periodontal disease in less affluent groups of patients.

Oral disorders such as periodontal disease imposes a significant burden on the individual affected, on society, nationally and globally. As current researchers delve into the task of re-quantifying periodontal diseases so that it encompasses the view of disease in a more absolute manner, we see an increasing interest in the use of patient-reported measures as an outcome of care (Aslund et al., 2008). In the following section, this chapter will look into the brief history on the development of such measures with regards to oral health and its current use in the field of periodontology.

4. Development of QoL Measures

Even with the vast amount of evidence flooding the dental field, the limitations in quantifying oral diseases is seen across all specialties. In periodontology, clinical indices and examinations such as the Basic Periodontal Examination, or even the routine periodontal charts, are essentially just measures of existing pathology or outcome of past oral diseases. To date, these clinical measures are still unable to tell us definitely whether a clinical finding such as an increased pocket depth is in fact a diseased entity or just a remnant of the destructive disease that once took place.

Most importantly, as the clinician strives by all means possible to eliminate this so called diseased periodontal pocket, the benefits of treatment may be minimal or even absent, making the morbidity due to such treatments on the patient unwarranted. Due to limitations in the traditional methods of quantifying disease, the concept of measuring and treating diseases has seen some changes over the years. Related concepts in health care have been redefined and a basic distinction drawn between disease and illness. Disease is often seen as a quantifiable deviation from certain physical, physiological or biochemical parameters such as blood counts, weight, height, and heart rate, accompanied by abnormalities in the structure or function of body organs or systems. Illness, however, is seen in a more personal context, being based largely on the patient's perspective of their own ill-health. It is a concept that is largely dependent upon their experience, social and cultural background as well as their personality traits (Helman, 1981).

An important point of departure from traditional methods of quantifying disease began with the definition of health offered by the WHO in 1948 as mentioned under section 3. With this, a conceptual framework on measuring health as not just a disease or pathological state but a multidimensional biophysical and socio-medical interaction was proposed by Locker (1988). Locker's concept was a simplified sequence of impacts or outcomes that were linked in a linear fashion to produce an overall scheme which moves from a biological to a behavioural and then social level of analysis. This model was an adaptation of that embraced by the WHO as part of the International Classification of Impairments, Disabilities and Handicaps (Locker, 1988).

Locker's suggested model (Figure 1) of measuring oral health draws upon the concepts of health defined by Wood (1980) in terms of impairment, functional limitation, disability and handicap. These identify distinct areas of human experience relative to disease and its personal and social consequences. It links concepts from both medicine and the behavioural sciences to capture a broad spectrum of events, each of which provides the basis for specific types of health status measure (Locker, 1988).

The categories and concepts of health as explained by Locker are discussed below.

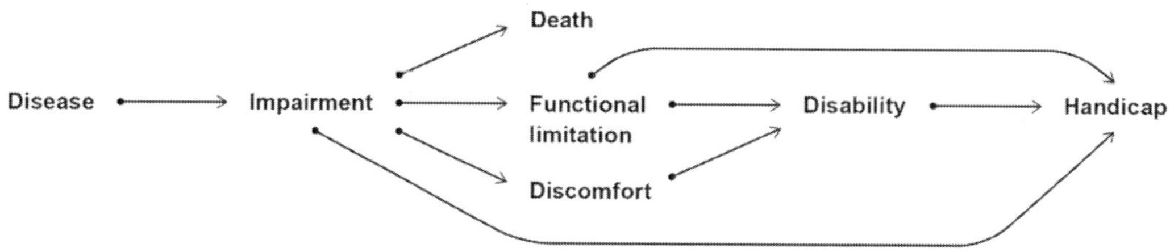

Figure 1. Modified WHO conceptual model of disease and psychosocial outcome by D. Locker, 1988, Community Dental Health 5, 3-18. Copyright 1988, BASCD. With permission.

4.1. Death

Death as an end-point of disease, though limited in its use with common oral diseases, is still an essential concept in assessing health (Locker, 1988). Although estimates of standardized mortality rates can still provide useful information on the impacts of diseases or treatment modalities, such comparisons for different diseases have become less meaningful in planning treatment. For example, in the case of cancers, most patients usually survive for more than 5–10 years, and thus one must wait for a long period of time for mortality to occur (Hung et al., 2014), and for obvious reasons, will not be popularly used as a desired outcome of treatment.

4.2. Disease

Disease in a more traditional sense has been described by Campbell et al., (1979):

> "A disease is the sum of the abnormal phenomena displayed by a group of living organisms in association with a specified common characteristic or set of characteristics by which they differ from the norm for their species in such a way as to place them at a biological disadvantage"

In Locker's model, disease was taken to be a label applied to the pathological processes and was measured in terms of its prevalence and incidence in populations. Sources of information may be from population surveys, cancer registrations, infectious disease reports or even hospital discharge forms (Locker, 1988).

4.3. Impairment

Impairment has been defined as any anatomical loss, structural abnormality or disturbances in physical or psychological processes, either present at birth or as a consequence of disease or injury (Locker, 1988). Such measures are commonly used in dentistry. Impairments are usually represented by traditional disease based indicators of oral health such as the DMFT index, or clinical attachment loss which as its name suggest, measures loss of periodontal attachment (Locker, 1988, Locker and Miller, 1994).

4.4. Functional Limitation

Functional limitations are defined as restrictions in the functions customarily expected of the body or its component organs or systems. In case of oral function, this would often refer to the ability to chew, eat and produce intelligible speech. Clinical measures of functional limitations are more ambiguous in nature, more difficult to evaluate and less common in dentistry (Locker, 1988, Locker and Miller, 1994).

4.5. Discomfort

The first three concepts of health mentioned above have often been regarded as the biophysical measures of health, referring more towards the biological consequences of disease itself (Locker, 1988). In the conceptual model by Locker, as it approaches the end of the continuum, health status measurements begin to merge with more subjective matters in relation to QoL. In this model, discomfort and pain were viewed together as a socio-medical measure because they are subjectively perceived and can be experienced even without any identifiable pathology or physiological dysfunction (Locker, 1988, Locker and Miller, 1994).

4.6. Disability

Disability refers to any difficulty performing activities of daily living. While traditional measures of disability focuses only on the physical restrictions one has, current health models view disabilities as a broader range of limitations in terms of physical, psychological and social function. Lockers conceptual model defines such limitations in terms of two components (Locker, 1988):

I. Physical well-being: Encompassing individual activity restrictions in such areas of life as mobility, self-care, eating, resting and so on.
II. Social well-being: Involving problems in the work place, at home and during recreation. Measures of social well-being include social integration, social contacts and social intimacy. The first is concerned with the extent of an individual's participation in community life. The second with the frequency of interaction with the community, and the third with the quality and emotional investment during such interactions.

4.7. Handicap

Handicap is defined as the disadvantage experienced by impaired and disabled people because they do not conform to the normalities set by society. While disability and functional limitations refer to the immediate personal consequences of disease, handicap is concerned with broader social effects (Locker, 1988). It is not a direct effect of the disease itself, but more of an indirect social consequence of disease. Any loss or abnormality of the structure or function or the behavioural limitations involved can be a disadvantage to the individual in terms of the quality of everyday life and long-term life chances. For instances, Tobiasen and Hiebert (1993) stated that children with facial clefts are at higher risk of reduced social competence such as development of friendships, progress in education, and participation in communal events leading to an overall negative effect on their psychosocial development (Tobiasen and Hiebert, 1993). Given the multidimensional effects of handicap, such disadvantages are difficult to quantify (Locker, 1988).

5. The Conceptual Model

The conceptual model by Locker illustrates the various relationships between the component parts of the overall model, linking each outcome of disease in a linear progression. At the end of the process, handicap may be seen as an outcome of sequential events starting from disease to impairment to functional limitation and eventually leading to life or social disadvantages. Furthermore, handicap may not be just an outcome of these series of events, but may be a direct consequence of impairment or functional limitations. Locker's model provides a theoretical framework for the empirical exploration of the relationships between different dimensions of disease and oral health (Locker and Miller, 1994). However, one inadequacy of the model was that there was no specific link from the defined health indicators to QoL (Locker, 2004). Wilson and Cleary (1995) proposed a model that makes an explicit link towards QoL. In their conceptual model, biological and physiological factors (or disease) result in symptoms, compromised physical and psychosocial functions and negative health perceptions leading towards a diminished QoL. As the model progresses from the basic biological and physiological concept of disease, its functional and psychosocial outcomes and its impact on QoL are said to be influenced by both individual and environmental characteristics. This concept moves the perception of health from a personal biological experience of the disease towards the impact it has on the individual as a member of society and vice versa. At the end of the process, QoL is also seen to be influenced by a wide range of non-medical factors such as work and education. Finally, the authors also clarified that the absence of connectors between different levels do not imply that no such relationships exist nor are any of the relationships unidirectional (Wilson and Cleary, 1995).

6. Changes in Assessment of Oral Health

Of recent years, as interest in the impact of oral health on the psychosocial profiles of patients continue to grow, oral health measures that draw on the patient's perspective previously referred to as socio-dental indicators, subjective oral health or the social impacts of oral disease were replaced with the term Oral Health-Related Quality of Life (OHRQoL) (Locker and Allen, 2007).

Referring back to the WHO (1995) definition of QOL as mentioned under section 1, OHRQoL characterizes a person's perception of how oral health influences their daily lives. OHRQoL is assessed specifically in terms of impact on physical, emotional and corresponding social functioning associated with performing normal roles brought about by each individual's oral state (McGrath and Bedi, 2001a, Ozcelik et al., 2007). To date, there is no consensus on a generally accepted definition of OHRQoL, but most authors are in agreement that it is a subjective construct best reported from a patient's point of view regarding their oral health and its effect on general well-being (Locker, 2004, Al-Harthi et al., 2013, Brauchle et al., 2013).

If a researcher aims to assess the OHRQoL of a specific group, then it is necessary to identify a measure whose items address various aspects of daily life that the target group in question considers important (Locker, 2004). Some of the most widely used generic OHRQoL instruments are: the Oral Health Impact Profile (OHIP) (Slade and Spencer, 1994); Oral Health-Related Quality of Life Measure (OHQoL-UK©) (McGrath and Bedi, 2001b); Oral Impacts on Daily Performance (OIDP) (Adulyanon et al., 1996) and the Geriatric Oral Health Assessment Index (GOHAI) (Atchison and Dolan, 1990), while condition-specific tools such as the Third Molar Health-Related Quality of Life instrument (Shugars et al., 1996); Orthognathic Quality of Life Questionnaire (OQLQ) (Cunningham et al., 2000); Dentine Hypersensitivity Experience Questionnaire (DHEQ) (Boiko et al., 2010) and the Halitosis Associated Life-quality Test (HALT) (Kizhner et al., 2011) are aimed at assessing the impact of specific oral problems on daily living. Though these measures differ in terms of their length, scoring systems and oral health concepts addressed, they all quantify OHRQoL in terms of numerical scores. These results can then be used to compare groups with and without oral disease, with disease at different stages and severity or different oral diseases. While the generic instruments are mainly used in assessing the overall impact of various oral problems on OHRQoL, the condition-specific questionnaires focuses on effects due to a single oral disease or problem. This makes the condition-specific instruments more sensitive to minor, but clinically important changes in specific oral diseases (Bernabe et al., 2009, Tsakos et al., 2010, Kizhner et al., 2011).

Most OHRQoL instruments have been tested for validity, internal consistency, reliability and responsiveness to change (Locker, 2004). Responsiveness refers to the ability of a measure to detect minimally important clinical changes. This allows such OHRQoL measures to detect small meaningful changes, both in-between groups and within-subject that occurs naturally or as a result of an intervention (Allen et al., 2001, Locker et al., 2004, Tsakos et al., 2010). As such, changes in OHRQoL measures can be assessed and compared in terms of their effect on patient reported psychosocial well-being before and after treatment (Locker, 2004). By using appropriate OHRQoL instruments, benefits of new, and usually expensive therapies such as dental implants may be assessed (Allen and Locker, 2002), providing both clinicians and policy makers more information when planning treatment and public health strategies (Allen et al., 2001, Locker, 2004). Of late, interest in measures of OHRQoL have been expanding in the field of periodontology and will be the topic of our next discussion.

7. Periodontal Disease and Oral Health-Related Quality of life (OHRQoL)

Periodontal disease has been described as an inflammatory condition initiated by bacterial complexes in the dental plaque biofilm. In the susceptible patient, advancing periodontal disease often leads to loss of both soft and hard tissues around teeth. Due to the nature and progression of the disease, methods of characterizing periodontal disease have often been focused on clinical parameters such as probing pockets depths and clinical attachment levels (Jansson et al., 2014). Unfortunately, such clinically based findings show no indication of how the disease affects the patients themselves. To date, little is known regarding this aspect of periodontal disease (Needleman et al., 2004, Wong et al., 2012). Obviously, such patients' daily lives are not going to be much affected by the knowledge of a few deep pockets in their mouth, neither is a high plaque score going to be of much significance to their usual routines. However, the consequences brought upon by signs and symptoms such as pain, discomfort, functional limitation and halitosis will have some sort of debilitating effect on their physical, social and psychological well-being (Needleman et al., 2004).

Periodontal disease has been shown to affect OHRQoL in patients. Patients often report functional limitation, physical pain and psychological disability associated with the disease. Needleman et al., (2004) assessed the impact of periodontal disease on the OHRQoL of 205 such patients attending a private specialist clinic over a 6 months period. Patients under various phases of periodontal treatment were evaluated using the OHQoL-UK© questionnaire. Sixteen key areas of OHRQoL as described by McGrath et al., (2000) were assessed, these were: symptoms of the disease such as comfort and bad breath; physical aspects such as eating, appearances, general health, speech and smiling or laughing; psychological aspects, which were relaxing, self-confidence, mood, being carefree and personality; social aspects in work, social life, finances and romance (McGrath et al., 2000). Responses to the OHQoL-UK© ranges from ''very bad'' (score 1) to ''very good'' (score 5) with lower score indicating poorer OHRQoL (McGrath et al., 2000, Needleman et al., 2004, Durham et al., 2013). Besides evaluating OHRQoL, patients were also asked to report about the signs and symptoms of periodontal disease in the past year, in terms of experiencing swollen, sore, or receding gums; loose teeth, drifting teeth, bad breath and toothache. The authors reported that the impact of periodontal disease on the subjects OHRQoL was considerable, with 90% of patients claiming that their OHRQoL was impacted by the signs and symptoms of the disease or its outcome in one way or more. A substantial number of patients reported bad or very bad effects on their OHRQoL. Of 205 subjects, 19% reported such effects (bad or very bad) on their comfort, 18% on bad breath, 18% on appearances, 16% on smiling or laughing, 32% on finances, 13% on their mood and 12% said periodontal disease detracted from their confidence. Patient's OHQoL-UK© scores were also significantly associated with self reported periodontal experiences of swollen, sore or receding gums, loose teeth and drifting teeth, bad breath and toothache, with patients self-reporting such signs and symptoms having worse OHRQoL than those who did not. Unsurprisingly, they also found that new patients had lower OHQoL-UK© scores indicative of diminished OHRQoL compared to those under periodontal maintenance, suggesting that periodontal therapy may improve OHRQoL. However a few limitations in this study could be observed. Firstly, the type of periodontal disease itself was not defined, secondly, no long term comparisons were made between treated and new patients, and no periodontally healthy subjects were included as controls. It would have been interesting to know if patients with either chronic or aggressive periodontitis would react differently due to the different rate of disease progression and the relatively early onset of the latter. Furthermore, it would be of importance to know how these patients fare before and after therapy, and if such patients do in fact have poorer OHRQoL compared to periodontally healthy subjects. Though not without its shortcomings, this study paved the way for a better understanding of how patients perceive the effects of periodontal disease and its outcome on their physical, psychological and social health.

A later report from the current group (Ng and Leung, 2006b) assessed the impact of periodontal health on OHRQoL in 1000 Chinese subjects in Hong Kong. Subjects were divided into a healthy/low periodontal attachment loss group (n = 584), and a high/severe periodontal attachment loss group (n = 143). It was reported that subjects with severe attachment loss perceived more functional limitation, physical pain, psychological discomfort, physical disability and psychological disability compared to their healthy counterparts. While prevalence of negative impact on the psychological domains of discomfort and disability varied between 4.0% and 6.3%, unfavourable effects on social disability and handicap was less prevalent. This was in slight contrast to the findings by Needleman et al., (2004). It was postulated that differences in cultural background and health beliefs may be the reasons accounting for such disparity. However, both reports concluded that subjects with better periodontal health were more likely to have better OHRQoL, and vice versa (Needleman et al., 2004, Ng and Leung, 2006b).

7.1. OHRQoL in Patients with Chronic Periodontitis

Chronic periodontitis (CP) is the most common form of periodontal disease predominantly seen in patients aged over 30. They usually present clinically with considerable amounts of plaque and calculus associated with marked gingival inflammation, periodontal pockets and attachment loss. In most cases, the disease progresses slowly though short periods of rapid periodontal destruction may occur. Although CP may be diagnosed as either a localized or generalized form, the two patterns of disease appear to be similar with regards to their pathogenesis and aetiology (Armitage, 1999).

CP impairs patient's OHRQoL (Wong et al., 2012, Brauchle et al., 2013, Durham et al., 2013, Jansson et al., 2014). A study by Durham et al., (2013) on 89 patients with CP using both the OHIP-49 and the OHQoL-UK© questionnaires concluded that patients OHRQoL were affected by signs and symptoms of the disease. In slight contrast to the OHQoL-UK© questionnaire, OHIP-49, as its name suggests, contains forty nine items, to which each response indicates the frequency of the impact on the individual, ranging from ''never'' (Score 0) to ''very often'' (Score 4). Summation of each response code generates both domain scores and an overall summary score with higher scores indicating poorer OHRQoL (Slade, 1998). Durham et al., (2013) reported that patients with chronic periodontitis had significantly poorer OHRQoL compared to periodontally healthy controls. Whether considering either OHIP-49 or OHQoL-UK©, the items with most statistically significant differences between patients with periodontitis and periodontally healthy subjects were related to reports of pain, halitosis, aesthetics and psychological concerns. These findings relate well with the results by Needleman et al., (2004), further strengthening the concept that periodontal disease negatively affects the OHRQoL of patients affected (Needleman et al., 2004, Ng and Leung, 2006b, Durham et al., 2013, Jansson et al., 2014).

When comparing the severity of periodontal disease and its impact on OHRQoL, Jansson and co-workers (2014) found that patients with a more severe form of CP reported poorer OHRQoL compared to patients with lesser radiographic bone loss. Using a shorter version of the OHIP questionnaire, OHIP-14, they evaluated the impact of periodontal disease on the OHRQoL between three groups of patients: patients with radiographic bone loss of less than one third of the root length (BL-), patients with radiographic bone loss of one third or more of the root length in <30% of teeth (BL), and patients with radiographic bone loss of one third or more of the root length in ≥30% of teeth (BL+). Patients from the third group (BL+) reported significantly worse OHRQoL compared with the other two, supporting a possible correlation between the degree of periodontal destruction and OHRQoL. They concluded that loss of clinical attachment and its severity may have an impact on patients' OHRQoL (Jansson et al., 2014).

It seems that from the currently available literature, CP impacts a patient in more ways than one. Not surprisingly, the consequences of disease such as pain, swelling, halitosis and ultimately tooth loss will affect the patient physically, psychologically and socially leading to a diminished OHRQoL.

7.2. OHRQoL in Patients with Aggressive Periodontitis

One of the less common and most severe forms of periodontal disease is aggressive periodontitis (AgP) which is characterized by a rapid rate of progression, early onset of disease and a tendency for familial aggregation. It typically presents itself in two forms- Localized AgP (LAgP) and Generalized AgP (GAgP).

Clinically, the signs and symptoms of the disease are extensive loss of supporting periodontal structures and bone resorption causing deep periodontal pockets, bleeding from the gingival sulcus, and tooth mobility eventually leading to tooth loss (Armitage, 1999, Armitage, 2004). LAgP has been known to be restricted to the first molars and incisors and reported to be self-arresting.

However, GAgP has more severe symptoms and individuals suffering from it experience considerable impact on their OHRQoL (Eltas and Uslu, 2013). Using the OHQoL-UK© instrument, Eltas and Uslu (2013) evaluated its association with GAgP patients' common complaints like missing teeth, recession, bleeding gums, halitosis, pain and tooth mobility and found that all complaints affected the OHQoL-UK© scores significantly. Deepest impact by GAgP on OHRQoL was on discomfort, eating enjoyment and breath odour. Finances, work and relaxation were least affected.

AgP negatively impacts patient's OHRQoL. Though further research is needed to compare such effects with that of CP and the general population, current evidence suggests that periodontal disease, regardless of its form, has significant deleterious outcomes on a patient's OHRQoL.

8. Impact of Periodontal Disease Sequelae on OHRQoL

8.1. Tooth Loss due to Periodontal Disease

The clinical signs and symptoms of periodontitis do not overtly affect the patient in the early stages of disease. However, the inadequately treated patient ultimately experiences tooth loss which would affect both, function and aesthetics depending on the number and position of tooth lost (Elias and Sheiham, 1998, Baba et al., 2008). Tooth loss may be a consequence of untreated periodontal disease or may be a part of periodontal therapy itself. Though both events may not affect patients OHRQoL differently, the impact of missing teeth within these two contexts will be discussed separately.

Several studies have been conducted to evaluate the impact of tooth loss on OHRQoL. Most have concluded that loss of teeth negatively impacts the OHRQoL of patients. Locker (1995) in his population study showed that after controlling other variables, OHIP score increased by 0.3 with each additional missing tooth. Similar results were reported by Steele and co-workers (2004). Batista et al., (2014), in their cross-sectional study, assessed the impact of tooth loss in 248 Brazilian adults aged 20 to 64 years old using the OHIP-14 questionnaire. Their analyses revealed a more severe impact on OHRQoL when the number of teeth lost was above 13. However, when at least one anterior tooth was missing, the severity of impact was higher than those with no or only posterior missing teeth, even when the total number of missing teeth was less than 13. Furthermore, low family income was associated with the prevalence of severe impact on OHRQoL (Batista et al., 2014).

When patients with periodontal disease are concerned, Durham et al., (2013) reported that patients with untreated chronic periodontitis perceived poorer OHRQoL in the domains of functional limitation, physical pain and overall OHIP-49 score due to tooth loss. They stated that increased missing teeth were associated with higher negative impacts of periodontitis on OHRQoL (Durham et al., 2013). Jansson et al., (2014) evaluated the periodontal condition of 443 subjects and found that number of remaining teeth had a statistically significant influence on subjects OHRQoL. Cunha-Cruz et al., (2007) stated that increased tooth loss was another clinical outcome of untreated periodontal patients associated with reduced OHRQoL and worse perceived oral health. Patients with ≥8 missing teeth reported being more self-conscious and experienced more denture discomfort (Cunha-Cruz et al., 2007). Similarly, Eltas and Uslu (2013) reported that as high as 85% of patients with untreated GAgP complaint of missing teeth. Moreover, such patients reported negative impacts on their comfort, eating/enjoyment of food, appearance, speech, general health, smiling/laughing, confidence, carefree manner, mood, personality, work/usual duties, romance and social life due to tooth loss (Eltas and Uslu, 2013).

When only posterior teeth are concerned, Käyser (1981) came to the conclusion that patients have enough capacity to adapt when a minimum of four occluding units are present (one unit equals to a pair of occluding premolars and two units equal to a pair of occluding molars). This concept was termed the shortened dental arches (Käyser, 1981). A literature review by Elias and Sheiham (1998) concluded that oral functional needs could be satisfied by a less than complete dentition. As such, though negative impacts of tooth loss on OHRQoL have been reported by patients with periodontal disease, the decision to restore or not to restore missing teeth is somewhat a subjective matter and will be discussed further down this chapter.

8.2. Gingivitis

Gingivitis is a reversible inflammatory response of the tooth-supporting tissues in response to bacterial biofilm. Though often considered a milder less-destructive condition of the periodontium, it can lead to uncomfortable consequences such as bleeding, swelling, enlargement, and pain depending on its severity. Moreover, the gingival margin forms an important part of a person's smile and it is obvious that any condition which impairs the aesthetics may have a negative impact on the OHRQoL. The effect of gingivitis on OHRQoL was found to be limited or insignificant in some studies (Chen and Hunter, 1996, Tsakos et al., 2006, Castro et al., 2011, Paula et al., 2012). However, in other studies such as the Thailand National Oral Health Survey on 12-15 year olds using the OIDP index, the authors reported a moderate to high impact of gingivitis on OHRQoL, especially in the psychological domain. Negative feelings towards smiling, academic achievements and making social interactions or low self image satisfaction resulting from gingivitis could affect the psychological health of children and adolescents (Krisdapong et al., 2012). Tomazoni and co-workers (2014) conducted a cross-sectional study to assess the child-OHRQoL (COHRQoL) in 12 year old Brazilian school children. They used the Child Perceptions Questionnaire for 11 to 14 year old children (CPQ11-14) which assesses COHRQoL using four subscales namely, oral symptoms, functional limitations, emotional well-being and social well-being. They found that extensive gingivitis had a greater impact on the children's self-perceived OHRQoL as compared to those with low levels or no gingivitis. Non-white children, females, children whose mothers did not complete primary education and those with low house hold income were found to have higher mean scores of CPQ11-14. The correlation between extensive gingivitis and CPQ11-14 scores was found mainly in the emotional domain which encompasses issues related to frustration or irritation, embarrassment, and concern about what other think about their teeth, lips or mouth (Tomazoni et al., 2014). Gingivitis in pregnancy is also found to have significantly negative impacts on the perceived OHRQoL. Acharya and co-workers (2009) conducted a cross-sectional study on 259 pregnant and 237 non-pregnant rural Indian women using the OHIP-14 questionnaire to compare the perceived OHRQoL in both groups. They found significantly higher mean number of sextants with CPITN scores of 2 and 3 and higher gingival index score in pregnant women compared to their non-pregnant counterparts. Concurrently, the perceived OHRQoL was also significantly poorer in pregnant women. They concluded that parity, DMFT scores and Gingival Index scores were significant predictors for OHRQoL (Acharya et al., 2009).

8.3. Periodontal Attachment Loss/ Marginal Bone Loss, Pain, Halitosis, Drifting of Teeth and Aesthetics

The clinical signs of periodontal disease such as 'clinical attachment loss (CAL)', 'probing pocket depth' and radiographic 'marginal bone loss' have been shown to be associated with OHRQoL in several studies. Recently, a few studies have also shown significant associations between the OHRQoL and patients' self-reported symptoms. In a study by our group (Ng and Leung, 2006b), subjects with mean full mouth CAL>3 mm were found to have significantly higher total mean Chinese OHIP short version (OHIP-14S) scores as compared to those with CAL $\leq$ 2 mm. Furthermore, there were also statistically significant differences in scores from five domains, which were functional limitation, physical pain, psychological discomfort, physical disability, and psychological disability between the two groups. There were significant associations between OHIP-14S scores and occurrence of self-reported 'swollen gums', 'sore gums', 'receding gums', 'loose teeth', 'bad breath', and 'toothache'. The symptom of 'drifting teeth' did not affect OHRQoL in this sample (Ng and Leung, 2006b).

Needleman et al., (2004) measured the impact of oral health on life quality using the OHQoL-UK© instrument. Their study sample included 205 patients attending a private periodontal clinic over 6 months. They found the OHQoL-UK© scores to be associated significantly with high number of PD$\geq$ 5mm with poorer life quality in such patients. Furthermore, unlike the previously mentioned study, all the self-reported symptoms, including 'drifting teeth' were significantly associated with poorer OHRQoL (Needleman et al., 2004).

Pain even in its mildest form most inevitably affects one's daily function. Saito's group (2010) reported a significant difference in experience of physical pain between individuals with or without periodontal disease at baseline. While Cunha-Cruz and colleagues (2007) stated that one of the three most commonly reported problems among untreated patients was pain. These observations suggest that not only the physical functioning, but also pleasurable life experiences, such as relaxation and social interaction, can be affected by the outcomes of periodontal disease.

Several other signs and symptoms of periodontal disease also have significant effects on patient's OHRQoL. Among others, halitosis or "breath-odour" was reported by several investigators (Needleman et al., 2004, Ng and Leung, 2006b, Durham et al., 2013, Eltas and Uslu, 2013) to negatively impact OHRQoL considerably. Halitosis is frequently experienced by patients and the most common causes originate from abnormalities in the oral cavity itself, namely tongue coating, periodontal disease, pharyngitis, laryngitis (Scully and Greenman, 2008).

With a high prevalence estimate of 20% to 34% (Liu et al., 2006, Bornstein et al., 2009) halitosis has a significant impact on the social and psychological health of the patient (Suzuki et al., 2008, Buunk-Werkhoven et al., 2012, He et al., 2012). A study by Zaitsu and co-workers (2011) revealed that 22.9% of patients with genuine halitosis defined as "obvious malodour with intensity beyond a socially acceptable level is perceived" (Yaegaki and Coil, 2000) were prone to general social anxiety disorder. Moreover, subjects at high risk of social anxiety disorder had difficulty in overcoming their anxiety about halitosis.

Similarly, possible aesthetic concerns arising from loss of interdental papilla (Cunha-Cruz et al., 2007) and missing anterior teeth (Cunha-Cruz et al., 2007, Al-Omiri et al., 2009, Gerritsen et al., 2010) may be driving the observed diminished OHRQoL and perceived poor oral health seen in patients with periodontal disease (Cunha-Cruz et al., 2007). Al Omiri and co-workers (2009) measured the Dental Impact on Daily living in 50 partially edentulous patients with missing anterior teeth and compared them with 50 control subjects with no missing teeth. They found significant correlations between number of missing anterior teeth and patient's satisfaction with appearance, oral comfort, general performance and eating dimensions. Higher number of missing teeth was associated with lower levels of satisfaction with dentition and daily living.

From the evidence available, the clinical presentations of periodontal disease which are readily perceivable by individuals, such as pain, tooth mobility, drifting of teeth, unaesthetic loss of interdental soft tissues and tooth loss (Cunha-Cruz et al., 2007) may eventually lead to psychosocial impacts. This is seen especially in severe and generalized forms of the disease, where patients may perceive a lack of confidence, inability to relax or feel carefree, poor mood and personality, while encountering problems with work, relationships and social interaction due to the biological effects of the disease (Eltas and Uslu, 2013). Furthermore, difficulties in eating, enjoying food, and other basic functions in daily life will also lead to worse general well-being (Ng and Leung, 2006b, Durham et al., 2013). These findings challenge the perception of periodontal disease as a silent disease (Cunha-Cruz et al., 2007). The relationships linking the biological outcomes of periodontal disease to physical, psychological and social consequences will be discussed further through a theoretical periodontal disease-OHRQoL model proposed later in this chapter.

9. Effects of Periodontal Therapy

9.1. Non-Surgical Periodontal Therapy and Its Impact on OHRQoL

Periodontal disease, be it chronic or aggressive in nature affects patients OHRQoL. Fortunately, recent studies have begun to show promising results that such effects on OHRQoL may diminish with proper treatment.

Initial periodontal therapy has a potential to improve OHRQoL. As mentioned in an earlier section, non-surgical periodontal therapy may ameliorate patient's signs and symptoms of periodontal disease and improve perceptions of oral health (Saito et al., 2010, Wong et al., 2012, Brauchle et al., 2013). This is seen especially in those with severe forms of the disease (Brauchle et al., 2013).

Saito and colleagues (2010) evaluated the change in OHRQoL after conventional non-surgical periodontal therapy in Japanese patients using the OHRQoL model for dental hygiene (OHRQL). Respondents were asked to answer questions related to seven domains namely pain, dry mouth, eating and chewing, speech, social function, psychological function and health perception with a lower frequency score suggesting better OHRQoL. They found significant improvements in most of the reported domains with greatest improvements observed in reports of pain (44% reduction in OHRQL score post treatment), followed by improvements in social function (31%), improvements in eating and chewing function (30%), while psychological domain showed moderate improvements (25%) (Saito et al., 2010).

Similarly Wong and colleagues (2012) showed that non-surgical periodontal therapy was associated with improved OHRQoL with regard to patient reported physical pain; psychological discomfort and disability 12 months post-treatment. They concluded that though periodontal attachment loss is somewhat irreversible, control of the disease and maintenance of its stability could have profound effects on patients at a more personal level. As discussed earlier, such observations reflect the need to view disease or illness in a more holistic manner and not allow clinician-determined parameters to take precedence over patient-centred outcomes as signs of improvement. The report suggested that to motivate patients towards receiving periodontal therapy and increase compliance towards proper maintenance, clinicians could stress upon the positive psychological OHRQoL effects of non-surgical periodontal treatment (Wong et al., 2012).

9.2. Surgical Periodontal Therapy and Its Impact on OHRQoL

There have been limited and varying conclusions regarding the benefits of surgical periodontal procedures on patients OHRQoL in the dental literature. This observation is not unusual as such treatment modalities exert significant pain, discomfort and morbidity at the initial phase of treatment and benefits may only be seen in the long run.

Tonetti and co-workers (2004) observed the initial healing events, post-treatment morbidity and patient perceptions of treatment outcomes of the papilla preservation flap with and without enamel matrix derivatives (EMD). They reported that only 24% of controls and 30% of tests (with EMD) reported some interference with their daily activities for an average of less than 4 days. At 12 months post-operatively, overall patient satisfaction for both test and control surgical groups was good. Patients reported improvements in ‘‘gum health” and the ‘‘ability to clean the treated area.” Most importantly, patients from both groups perceived better oral health in terms of preserving their teeth and improvements in chewing ability (Tonetti et al., 2004). Ozcelik et al., (2007) evaluated the immediate post-operative effects of non-surgical (NS) periodontal treatment, flap surgery (SG) alone and flap surgery with enamel matrix derivatives (S+EMD) on the OHRQoL of patients treated. Patients' OHRQoL were assessed with the GOHAI and OHIP-14 questionnaires and followed up daily up to 7 days after therapy. They found that patients treated by surgery alone reported worse OHRQoL in terms of increased functional limitations, increased pain and discomfort, more psychological and behavioural impacts compared to the NS and S+EMD groups (Ozcelik et al., 2007). The Saito group (2011) followed up their patients 3-4 months after surgery and found no significant differences in patients' OHRQoL between post-initial therapy and post-surgery intervals. They suggested that during the course of periodontal treatment, non-surgical therapy relieves patient's signs and symptoms of the disease to an extent that any further improvements in OHRQoL would no longer be significantly reflected after surgical treatment (Saito et al., 2011). From the evidence discussed, it would be justified to state that adequate periodontal therapy helps diminish the negative effects of periodontal disease on OHRQoL. However, a further look into the literature shows that the outcome of different treatment strategies have, to varying degrees, an effect on patients OHRQoL as well. This is indeed true to the fact that comprehensive periodontal care which involves non-surgical and surgical therapy, extractions and even rehabilitative procedures will have both positive and negative implications on the patient's daily life.

9.3. Dentine Hypersensitivity and Its Impact on OHRQoL

Regardless of the type of periodontal therapy carried out, such therapeutic measures are not without complications. One such complication is pain. Pihlstrom and colleagues (1999) used the Heft-Parker pain scale in 52 adults with moderate periodontitis to evaluate pre and post- scaling and root planning pain. They reported that pain after such treatment was maximal between two to eight hours, lasted for six hours and then returned to pre-treatment pain levels on the next day (Pihlstrom et al., 1999).

As continuous severe pain after therapy would suggest incomplete treatment, it would not be considered in this discussion. However, one of the most common complaints reported among patients after periodontal treatment is pain in the form of dentine hypersensitivity (Rees et al., 2003, Tonetti et al., 2004). Dentine hypersensitivity has been reported to occur in approximately 50%-98% of patients after periodontal treatment (Chabanski et al., 1997, von Troil et al., 2002, Lin and Gillam, 2012). Denuded tooth surfaces leading to exposed dentine appears to be the major cause of dentine hypersensitivity (Dowell and Addy, 1983), as such, the high prevalence of dentine hypersensitivity among treated patients is somewhat expected as gingival recession (von Troil et al., 2002) and removal of root cementum leading to exposure of dentine are common complications of periodontal procedures (Jones et al., 1972, Ritz et al., 1991).

When comparing non-surgical and surgical periodontal therapy, postoperative sensitivity was found to be higher among patients after surgical procedures. Patients who had undergone flap surgery and osseous re-contouring were reported to have a high degree of discomfort probably due to increased treatment time, exposure of bone and more root surfaces (Lin and Gillam, 2012). Studies on the effects of dentine hypersensitivity on OHRQoL are severely lacking (Boiko et al., 2010, Lin and Gillam, 2012, Bekes and Hirsch, 2013). One study by Bekes et al., (2009) comparing OHRQoL impairment in patients seeking treatment for hypersensitive teeth in comparison with the general population found that most patients seeking treatment for dentine hypersensitivity were often limited in their eating, drinking and oral hygiene habits. They also showed that patients complaining of sensitive teeth reported substantial impairment in their OHRQoL (Bekes et al., 2009, Bekes and Hirsch, 2013).

Though current evidence is limited, it does show that dentine hypersensitivity may have a negative impact on OHRQoL among patients treated for periodontal disease. While the magnitude of effect may only be mild to moderate (Lin and Gillam, 2012), dentine hypersensitivity remains a challenge to the clinician due to its high prevalence among such patients.

9.4. Tooth Loss after Therapy and OHRQoL

Extraction of teeth is sometimes inevitable in patients with periodontal disease. Even treated patients with reasonably good initial treatment outcomes are at risk of further tooth loss (Hirschfeld and Wasserman, 1978, Tonetti et al., 2000, Leung et al., 2006).

Tonetti et al., (2000) evaluated 273 patients who had completed a full range of periodontal and restorative treatment and were placed under supervised supportive periodontal care. They reported that even with strict maintenance, 41% of patients had lost one or more teeth during recall. They also found that progressing periodontal disease was the major factor associated with tooth loss in this population with 57% of extracted teeth being lost due to severe periodontitis.

This group (Leung et al., 2006) retrospectively assessed the pattern of tooth loss in 97 Chinese subjects who had favourable responses to periodontal treatment done in a teaching hospital. These patients were discharged upon completing treatment and were responsible for their own dental care and periodontal maintenance. It was found that the annualized tooth loss rate for such patients was 0.25 teeth per patient per year, with upper molars and first premolars, lower second molars and incisors more prone to loss. Furthermore, continuing smokers, elderly patients, those wearing removable partial dentures, those with lower education levels or not performing inter-dental cleaning were found to be more susceptible to further periodontal breakdown and should be targeted for a strict hospital-clinic-based maintenance regime (Leung et al., 2006).

As discussed earlier, tooth loss affects OHRQoL in patients (Gerritsen et al., 2010, Zhang et al., 2013). However, it may seem that the replacement of such loss may not be essential in improving or maintaining one's OHRQoL (Elias and Sheiham, 1998, Tan et al., 2014).

As mentioned earlier, Käyser's group concluded that at least four posterior occlusal units preferably in a symmetrical position were sufficient to maintain adequate oral function in shortened dental arches (Käyser, 1981, Witter et al., 1990, Kalk et al., 1993). Further studies by this group went on to show that clinically there were no significant differences in subjects with three to five occluding units as compared to those with a complete dentition with respect to chewing ability, swallowing, temporomandibular joint disorders, tooth migration, periodontal support and oral comfort (Witter et al., 1987, Witter et al., 1990, Witter et al., 1991, Witter et al., 1994, Sarita et al., 2003, Kanno and Carlsson, 2006, Kreulen et al., 2012, Gerritsen et al., 2013). Restoration of molar occlusion with removable partial dentures did not appear to improve patient perceived function and may even worsen it (Käyser et al., 1987, Witter et al., 1989, Kalk et al., 1993).

Gerritsen and colleagues (2010) reviewed the impact of tooth loss on OHRQoL. They stated that the number of occluding pairs of teeth is important in predicting patient's OHRQoL, and that OHRQoL drops sharply only when the numbers of teeth present falls below 20. As patients with a shortened dental arch do not seem to have poorer OHRQoL, they suggested that application of the shortened dental arch approach be considered particularly in older adults. Such a strategy may help reduce financial burden on society as oral health care with an intervention led focus is expensive, and demand for this care, though not necessarily beneficial, may increase as society ages (Gerritsen et al., 2010).

Tan et al., (2014) stated that Australians with four occlusal units and intact anterior teeth reported equivalent OHRQoL to those who retained more natural teeth. They concluded that since OHRQoL among people with shortened dental arches was not inferior to that of people with more natural teeth, treatment goals should be changed from the costly rehabilitation of complete dental arches towards the preservation of a reduced, natural and functional dentition (Tan et al., 2014).

Though the maintenance of a shortened dental arch seems like a reasonable aim for the aging population, position of missing teeth, social and psychological values all have an effect on the OHRQoL of patients with tooth loss (Elias and Sheiham, 1998, Baba et al., 2008, Gerritsen et al., 2010, Zhang et al., 2013, Sukumar et al., 2015). Baba and colleagues (2008) showed that Japanese patients attending six prosthodontic clinics who lost only second molar contacts exhibited significantly better OHRQoL than those who lost more teeth. They concluded that patterns of missing occlusal units are likely to be related to OHRQoL impairment. The presence of first molar contacts may have an important role in determining OHRQoL in certain groups of patients (Baba et al., 2008). Gerritsen et al., (2010) reported that subjects with at least one missing anterior tooth were 1.8 times more likely to report an impact on their daily life. While Sukumar et al., (2015) found that patients reported greater OHRQoL improvement in terms of function and aesthetics when both posterior and anterior missing teeth were replaced.

As OHRQoL is an extremely subjective measure, it seems that the decision to restore or not to restore missing teeth may be dependent upon the population of patient being treated. Moreover, the type of restorative treatment carried out may also influence the satisfaction of each patient in terms of improvements in OHRQoL and will be briefly discussed.

9.5. Oral Rehabilitation and OHRQoL

Prosthodontic rehabilitation is a heterogeneous group of treatments which may be distinguished by location of treatment (anterior or posterior), type of replacements (fix or removable) and type of denture-bearing structure (implant, tooth, mucosa) (Sukumar et al., 2015). Restoration of missing teeth affects both function and appearance. Generally, it may be regarded that treatment in the anterior spaces will mainly affect aesthetics while restoration of posterior spaces will mostly affect function. Each of these dimensions, individually or added together, would have a significant contribution to the one's overall OHRQoL (John et al., 2004, Pavel et al., 2012, Montero et al., 2013, Yu et al., 2013, Misumi et al., 2014, Aarabi et al., 2015, Sukumar et al., 2015). John et al., (2004) assessed the change in OHRQoL of patient receiving fixed dental prosthesis (FDP), removable partial dental prosthesis (RDP) and complete dentures (CD). They found significantly improved OHRQoL measures in all treatment groups post-therapy with slightly better outcome in FDP versus RDP and CD. Similarly, Montero et al., (2012) evaluated the OHRQoL of patients receiving fixed dental prosthesis (FDP), metal based removable partial dentures (M-RPDs), acrylic removable partial dentures (ADs) and complete dentures (CDs) before and one month after treatment. They reported significant improvements in OHIP-14 domain scores in terms of chewing ability, smile aesthetics and satisfaction with the state of the mouth for all treatment groups. FDPs were reported to be more comfortable than ADs, while M-RPDs provided significantly better improvements in terms of ease of oral hygiene and partner relations, compared to FDPs. Patients receiving FDPs also reported slightly better eating comfort compared to other types of dental prosthesis (Montero et al., 2013). Similarly Aarabi and co-workers (2015) reported that conventional prosthodontic treatment with either fixed or removable dental prosthesis and complete dentures all yielded significant improvements in terms of OHRQoL measures with detectable treatment effects lasting up to two years. Of recent years, osseointegrated dental implants have become a widely acceptable means of replacing individual tooth, or as abutments for both fix and removable prosthesis. Studies by various authors on the different uses of dental implants have shown good treatment outcomes in terms of OHRQoL (Thomason et al., 2007, Pavel et al., 2012, Yu et al., 2013, Misumi et al., 2014, Oh et al., 2014). Thomason and colleagues (2007) reported that patients were more satisfied with implant-supported overdentures than conventional complete dentures and there was strong evidence that OHRQoL can be significantly improved using implant-supported overdentures. Similarly, Oh et al., (2014) concluded that implant-supported overdentures improved OHRQoL in patients with edentulous maxilla, mandible, or both, irrespective of the type of prosthesis provided (fixed or removable) compared to complete dentures. OHRQoL dimensions of functional limitation, physical pain, psychological discomfort, and psychological disability in the fixed prosthesis group, and functional limitation in the removable prosthesis group showed significant improvements compared to the complete denture group (Oh et al., 2014). In terms of implant treatment in the aesthetic area, Yu et al., (2013) showed that patients having their removable dentures replaced with implants in the anterior spaces perceived better OHRQoL after treatment. Significant improvements in terms of disability, psychological discomfort, functional limitation, pain, and discomfort were observed after implant therapy was completed (Yu et al., 2013). From the evidence presented, patient's OHRQoL may be improved when missing teeth are being replaced. Though different prosthodontic options have been shown to exert positive effects on overall OHRQoL, fixed options or treatment with dental implants seems to have a tendency for better improvements.

10. Adapted Model Linking Periodontal Disease and OHRQoL

From the discussion so far, periodontal disease does in fact impact OHRQoL. Treatment of the disease also affects OHRQoL. Such changes in OHRQoL may very well influence the disease itself, as well as affect each individual's systemic health and vice versa. As such, a proposed model linking periodontal disease, OHRQoL and other associated factors seems appropriate (Figure 2).

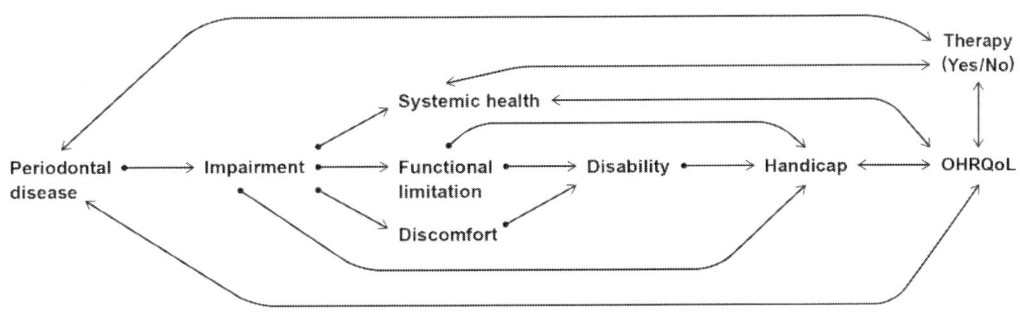

Figure 2. Adapted periodontal disease-OHRQoL model. Modified from D. Locker, 1988, Community Dental Health 5, 3-18. Copyright 1988, BASCD. Adapted with permission.

From Locker's adapted model it was explained that the biological outcome of disease can lead to social disadvantages whereby patient's life chances may be affected due to the limitations he/she suffers as a consequence of disease. This series of events, though not necessarily taking place in a consecutive manner will impact patient's OHRQoL. From a periodontal disease point of view, patient's self perceived OHRQoL may inherently affect the way he/she feels about the consequences of disease i.e. impairment, functional limitation, discomfort, disability and handicap, leading to a change in emotions, behaviours, stress level, coping mechanisms and ultimately a change in the presentation and outcome of disease. The present group (Ng and Leung, 2006a) showed that high/severe attachment loss was significantly associated with work strain, financial strain and depression. Those with high levels of job strain or financial strain with less favourable personality dispositions, determined from high scores of anxiety trait or depression trait, experienced more severe periodontal tissue destruction. Conversely, those with low scores of anxiety trait or depression trait, had less periodontal attachment loss, even though job strain or financial strain was high (Ng and Leung, 2006a). As such, a two way relationship between one's self perceived OHRQoL and periodontal disease should exists.

As discussed previously, various treatment strategies for patients with periodontal disease have undoubtedly some effects on the patients' OHRQoL and are shown in the current adapted model. Furthermore, patients without treatment may experience a change in periodontal disease status, leading towards a chronic cycle of events, with each cycle impacting the patient's biological, psychological and social function in a different way, leading to a further change in self-perceived OHRQoL.

In periodontal disease, death is not a likely outcome. However, relationships between periodontal disease, systemic health and OHRQoL are possible (de Pinho et al., 2012, Cicciu et al., 2013, Huang et al., 2013, Lindenmeyer et al., 2013). Due to the inflammatory nature of periodontal disease, treatment strategies or even absence of treatment may improve or worsen systemic health (Simpson et al., 2010, Chapple and Genco, 2013, Tonetti and Van Dyke, 2013, Jeffcoat et al., 2014), and is represented in the two-way arrow between therapy and systemic health. For example, treatment of periodontal disease is shown to improve glycaemic control in diabetic patients, and its effect is similar to adding a second diabetic drug (Chapple and Genco, 2013).

Rationally speaking, such improvements would affect the patient's general QoL and OHRQoL, though further research is warranted. Jeffcoat et al., (2014) found that patients with periodontitis with either type-2 diabetes; coronary artery disease; cerebral vascular disease or pregnancy, incurred lower medical costs and hospitalizations after they received periodontal therapy compared to untreated controls. In each case, the difference was statistically significant and involved considerable finances (11%–74% lower in the treated group) (Jeffcoat et al., 2014). Though such interventional efficacy of periodontal therapy on systemic health is far from solid, these findings suggest a plausible link between periodontal disease; its treatment and systemic health. These will all possibly affect one's OHRQoL as pointed out in the periodontal disease-OHRQoL model.

From the adapted model, though not marked by interconnecting arrows, both direct and indirect relationships can exist between individual outcomes of periodontal disease and OHRQoL. Such relationships can be seen in previously discussed evidence where tooth loss, severe marginal bone loss and pockets ≥5 mm were found to be associated with negative impacts on OHRQoL (Needleman et al., 2004, Cunha-Cruz et al., 2007, Durham et al., 2013, Jansson et al., 2014). Though not specifically shown in the model, these findings suggest a link between impairment (anatomical loss or structural abnormality) caused by periodontal disease on one's OHRQoL.

Another possible consequence of periodontal destruction (impairment) is reduction in periodontal support around teeth, increased mobility and pain (functional limitation and discomfort), and subsequently difficulty in eating (disability) leading towards an inability to enjoy societal interactions (handicap). Such sequences of events draw attention to the influence of periodontal disease on daily activities and its negative impact on overall OHRQoL (Ng and Leung, 2006b). Similarly when tooth loss, especially in the anterior region is concerned, individuals affected may experience social handicap in the form of diminished life chances such as employment or romance. Such a relationship between tooth loss and sociology is by all means possible (Rousseau et al., 2014).

Conclusion

Periodontal disease negatively affects one's OHRQoL and the extent of impact is correlated with the severity of periodontal disease (Needleman et al., 2004, Ng and Leung, 2006a, Ng and Leung, 2006b, Aslund et al., 2008, de Pinho et al., 2012, Shanbhag et al., 2012, Brauchle et al., 2013, Durham et al., 2013, Jansson et al., 2014). The treatment of periodontal disease itself has varying consequences on patients physiological, psychological and social well-being, leading to a change in overall OHRQoL (Needleman et al., 2004, Tonetti et al., 2004, Saito et al., 2010&2011, Lin and Gillam, 2012, Shanbhag et al., 2012, Wong et al., 2012, Jeffcoat et al., 2014). Furthermore, patients are able to better relate disease and treatment with self-reported outcomes measures such as OHRQoL than surrogate markers such as probing pocket depth and clinical attachment loss. Knowledge of OHRQoL can potentially motivate patients to improve adherence to oral health practices and increase compliance with maintenance therapy (Shanbhag et al., 2012, Wong et al., 2012). These factors are crucial for the long-term success of periodontal treatment.

Though the multidirectional relationships between the outcomes of periodontal disease, its treatment, systemic health and the disease itself may be oversimplified in the periodontal disease-OHRQoL model suggested, such a model may prove useful in guiding future research on this subject. Links between each proposed parameter in the model may be further clarified through well-conducted trials. Indeed, to truly understand and conceptualized the effects of periodontal disease on OHRQoL, further well-designed longitudinal studies are required. Future research should evaluate long term OHRQoL changes in patients receiving different forms of periodontal and/or restorative therapy. Moreover, the impacts of such treatments on OHRQoL in patients with different forms and severities of periodontal disease and in those with associated systemic conditions also deserve further exploration (Shanbhag et al., 2012).

Acknowledgments

The work described in this chapter was partially supported by a grant from the Research Grants Council of the Hong Kong Special Administrative Region, China (HKU 772110M).

References

[1] Aarabi, G., John, M. T., Schierz, O., Heydecke, G. & Reissmann, D. R. (2015) The course of prosthodontic patients' oral health-related quality of life over a period of 2 years. *Journal of Dentistry* 43, 261-268.

[2] Acharya, S., Bhat, P. V. & Acharya, S. (2009) Factors affecting oral health-related quality of life among pregnant women. *International Journal of Dental Hygiene* 7, 102-107.

[3] Adulyanon, S., Vourapukjaru, J. & Sheiham, A. (1996) Oral impacts affecting daily performance in a low dental disease Thai population. *Community Dentistry and Oral Epidemiology* 24, 385-389.

[4] Al-Harthi, L. S., Cullinan, M. P., Leichter, J. W. & Thomson, W. M. (2013) The impact of periodontitis on oral health-related quality of life: a review of the evidence from observational studies. *Australian Dental Journal* 58, 274-277; quiz 384.

[5] Al-Omiri, M. K., Karasneh, J. A., Lynch, E., Lamey, P. J. & Clifford, T. J. (2009) Impacts of missing upper anterior teeth on daily living. *International Dental Journal* 59, 127-132.

[6] Allen, F. & Locker, D. (2002) A modified short version of the oral health impact profile for assessing health-related quality of life in edentulous adults. *International Journal of Prosthodontics* 15, 446-450.

[7] Allen, P. F., McMillan, A. S. & Locker, D. (2001) An assessment of sensitivity to change of the Oral Health Impact Profile in a clinical trial. *Community Dentistry and Oral Epidemiology* 29, 175-182.

[8] Antunes, J. L., Pegoretti, T., de Andrade, F. P., Junqueira, S. R., Frazao, P. & Narvai, P. C. (2003) Ethnic disparities in the prevalence of dental caries and restorative dental treatment in Brazilian children. *International Dental Journal* 53, 7-12.

[9] Armitage, G. C. (1999) Development of a classification system for periodontal diseases and conditions. *Annals of Periodontology* 4, 1-6.

[10] Armitage, G. C. (2004) Periodontal diagnoses and classification of periodontal diseases. *Periodontology 2000* 34, 9-21.

[11] Aslund, M., Pjetursson, B. E. & Lang, N. P. (2008) Measuring oral health-related quality-of-life using OHQoL-GE in periodontal patients presenting at the University of Berne, Switzerland. *Oral Health and Preventive Dentistry* 6, 191-197.

[12] Atchison, K. A. & Dolan, T. A. (1990) Development of the Geriatric Oral Health Assessment Index. *Journal of Dental Education* 54, 680-687.

[13] Baba, K., Igarashi, Y., Nishiyama, A., John, M. T., Akagawa, Y., Ikebe, K., Ishigami, T., Kobayashi, H. & Yamashita, S. (2008) Patterns of missing occlusal units and oral health-related quality of life in SDA patients. *Journal of Oral Rehabilitation* 35, 621-628.

[14] Bagramian, R. A., Garcia-Godoy, F. & Volpe, A. R. (2009) The global increase in dental caries. A pending public health crisis. *AmeriCan. J.ournal of Dentistry* 22, 3-8.

[15] Batista, M., Lawrence, H. & Rosario de Sousa, M. (2014) Impact of tooth loss related to number and position on oral health quality of life among adults. *Health and Quality of Life Outcomes* 12, 165.

[16] Bekes, K. & Hirsch, C. (2013) What is known about the influence of dentine hypersensitivity on oral health-related quality of life? *Clinical Oral Investigations* 17 Suppl 1, S45-51.

[17] Bekes, K., John, M. T., Schaller, H. G. & Hirsch, C. (2009) Oral health-related quality of life in patients seeking care for dentin hypersensitivity. *Journal of Oral Rehabilitation* 36, 45-51.

[18] Bernabe, E., de Oliveira, C. M., Sheiham, A. & Tsakos, G. (2009) Comparison of the generic and condition-specific forms of the Oral Impacts on Daily Performances (OIDP) Index. *Journal of Public Health Dentistry* 69, 176-181.

[19] Boiko, O. V., Baker, S. R., Gibson, B. J., Locker, D., Sufi, F., Barlow, A. P. & Robinson, P. G. (2010) Construction and validation of the quality of life measure for dentine hypersensitivity (DHEQ). *Journal of Clinical Periodontology* 37, 973-980.

[20] Bornstein, M. M., Kislig, K., Hoti, B. B., Seemann, R. & Lussi, A. (2009) Prevalence of halitosis in the population of the city of Bern, Switzerland: a study comparing self-reported and clinical data. *European Journal of Oral Sciences* 117, 261-267.

[21] Brauchle, F., Noack, M. & Reich, E. (2013) Impact of periodontal disease and periodontal therapy on oral health-related quality of life. *International Dental Journal* 63, 306-311.

[22] Buunk-Werkhoven, Y., Dijkstra-le Clercq, M., Verheggen-Udding, E., de Jong, N. & Spreen, M. (2012) Halitosis and oral health-related quality of life: a case report. *International Journal of Dental Hygiene* 10, 3-8.

[23] Campbell, E. J., Scadding, J. G. & Roberts, R. S. (1979) The concept of disease. *British Medical Journal* 2, 757-762.

[24] Castro R. A., Portela, M. C., Leao, A. T. & de Vasconcellos, M. T. (2011) Oral health-related quality of life of 11- and 12-year-old public school children in Rio de Janeiro. *Community Dentistry and Oral Epidemiology* 39, 336-344.

[25] Chabanski, M. B., Gillam, D. G., Bulman, J. S. & Newman, H. N. (1997) Clinical evaluation of cervical dentine sensitivity in a population of patients referred to a specialist periodontology department: a pilot study. *Journal of Oral Rehabilitation* 24, 666-672.

[26] Chapple, I. L. & Genco, R. (2013) Diabetes and periodontal diseases: consensus report of the Joint EFP/AAP Workshop on Periodontitis and Systemic Diseases. *Journal of Clinical Periodontology* 40 Suppl 14, S106-112.

[27] Chen, M. S. & Hunter, P. (1996) Oral health and quality of life in New Zealand: a social perspective. *Social Science and Medicine* 43, 1213-1222.

[28] Cicciu, M., Matacena, G., Signorino, F., Brugaletta, A., Cicciu, A. & Bramanti, E. (2013) Relationship between oral health and its impact on the quality life of Alzheimer's disease patients: a supportive care trial. *International Journal of Clinical and Experimental Medicine* 6, 766-772.

[29] Cunha-Cruz, J., Hujoel, P. P. & Kressin, N. R. (2007) Oral health-related quality of life of periodontal patients. *Journal of Periodontal Research* 42, 169-176.

[30] Cunningham, S. J., Garratt, A. M. & Hunt, N. P. (2000) Development of a condition-specific quality of life measure for patients with dentofacial deformity: I. Reliability of the instrument. *Community Dentistry and Oral Epidemiology* 28, 195-201.

[31] de Pinho, A. M., Borges, C. M., de Abreu, M. H., EF, E. F. & Vargas, A. M. (2012) Impact of periodontal disease on the quality of life of diabetics based on different clinical diagnostic criteria. *International Journal of Dentistry* 2012, 986412.

[32] Dowell, P. & Addy, M. (1983) Dentine hypersensitivity--a review. Aetiology, symptoms and theories of pain production. *Journal of Clinical Periodontology* 10, 341-350.

[33] Durham, J., Fraser, H. M., McCracken, G. I., Stone, K. M., John, M. T. & Preshaw, P. M. (2013) Impact of periodontitis on oral health-related quality of life. *Journal of Dentistry* 41, 370-376.

[34] Elias, A. C. & Sheiham, A. (1998) The relationship between satisfaction with mouth and number and position of teeth. *Journal of Oral Rehabilitation* 25, 649-661.

[35] Eltas, A. & Uslu, M. O. (2013) Evaluation of oral health-related quality-of-life in patients with generalized aggressive periodontitis. *Acta Odontologica Scandinavica* 71, 547-552.

[36] Flemmig, T. F. & Beikler, T. (2013) Economics of periodontal care: market trends, competitive forces and incentives. *Periodontology 2000* 62, 287-304.

[37] Gerritsen, A. E., Allen, P. F., Witter, D. J., Bronkhorst, E. M. & Creugers, N. H. (2010) Tooth loss and oral health-related quality of life: a systematic review and meta-analysis. *Health and Quality of Life Outcomes* 8, 126.

[38] Gerritsen, A. E., Witter, D. J., Bronkhorst, E. M. & Creugers, N. H. (2013) An observational cohort study on shortened dental arches--clinical course during a period of 27-35 years. *Clinical Oral Investigations* 17, 859-866.

[39] Gift, H. C., Reisine, S. T. & Larach, D. C. (1992) The social impact of dental problems and visits. *AmeriCan. J.ournal of Public Health* 82, 1663-1668.

[40] He, S. L., Wang, J. H., Wang, M. H. & Deng, Y. M. (2012) Validation of the Chinese version of the Halitosis Associated Life-quality Test (HALT) questionnaire. *Oral Diseases* 18, 707-712.

[41] Helman, C. G. (1981) Disease versus illness in general practice. *Journal of the Royal College of General Practitioners* 31, 548-552.

[42] Hirschfeld, L. & Wasserman, B. (1978) A long-term survey of tooth loss in 600 treated periodontal patients. *Journal of Periodontology* 49, 225-237.

[43] Hosseinpoor, A. R., Itani, L. & Petersen, P. E. (2012) Socio-economic inequality in oral healthcare coverage: results from the World Health Survey. *Journal of Dental Research* 91, 275-281.

[44] Huang, D. L., Chan, K. C. & Young, B. A. (2013) Poor oral health and quality of life in older U.S. adults with diabetes mellitus. *Journal of the American Geriatrics Society* 61, 1782-1788.

[45] Hung, M., Lai, W., Chen, H. H., Su, W. & Wang, J. (2014) Comparison of expected health impacts for major cancers: Integration of incidence rate and loss of quality-adjusted life expectancy. *Cancer Epidemiology*.

[46] Jansson, H., Wahlin, A., Johansson, V., Akerman, S., Lundegren, N., Isberg, P. E. & Norderyd, O. (2014) Impact of periodontal disease experience on oral health-related quality of life. *Journal of Periodontology* 85, 438-445.

[47] Jeffcoat, M. K., Jeffcoat, R. L., Gladowski, P. A., Bramson, J. B. & Blum, J. J. (2014) Impact of periodontal therapy on general health: evidence from insurance data for five systemic conditions. *AmeriCan. J.ournal of Preventive Medicine* 47, 166-174.

[48] John, M. T., Slade, G. D., Szentpetery, A. & Setz, J. M. (2004) Oral health-related quality of life in patients treated with fixed, removable, and complete dentures 1 month and 6 to 12 months after treatment. *International Journal of Prosthodontics* 17, 503-511.

[49] Jones, S. J., Lozdan, J. & Boyde, A. (1972) Tooth surfaces treated in situ with periodontal instruments. Scanning electron microscopic studies. *British Dental Journal* 132, 57-64.
[50] Kalk, W., Käyser, A. F. & Witter, D. J. (1993) Needs for tooth replacement. *International Dental Journal* 43, 41-49.
[51] Kanno, T. & Carlsson, G. E. (2006) A review of the shortened dental arch concept focusing on the work by the Kayser/Nijmegen group. *Journal of Oral Rehabilitation* 33, 850-862.
[52] Käyser, A. F. (1981) Shortened dental arches and oral function. *Journal of Oral Rehabilitation* 8, 457-462.
[53] Käyser, A. F., Witter, D. J. & Spanauf, A. J. (1987) Overtreatment with removable partial dentures in shortened dental arches. *Australian Dental Journal* 32, 178-182.
[54] Kizhner, V., Xu, D. & Krespi, Y. P. (2011) A new tool measuring oral malodor quality of life. *European Archives of Oto-Rhino-Laryngology* 268, 1227-1232.
[55] Kreulen, C. M., Witter, D. J., Tekamp, F. A., Slagter, A. P. & Creugers, N. H. (2012) Swallowing threshold parameters of subjects with shortened dental arches. *Journal of Dentistry* 40, 639-643.
[56] Krisdapong, S., Prasertsom, P., Rattanarangsima, K., Sheiham, A. & Tsakos, G. (2012) The impacts of gingivitis and calculus on Thai children's quality of life. *Journal of Clinical Periodontology* 39, 834-843.
[57] Leung, W. K., Ng, D. K., Jin, L. & Corbet, E. F. (2006) Tooth loss in treated periodontitis patients responsible for their supportive care arrangements. *Journal of Clinical Periodontology* 33, 265-275.
[58] Lin, Y. H. & Gillam, D. G. (2012) The prevalence of root sensitivity following periodontal therapy: a systematic review. *International Journal of Dentistry* 2012, 407023.
[59] Lindenmeyer, A., Bowyer, V., Roscoe, J., Dale, J. & Sutcliffe, P. (2013) Oral health awareness and care preferences in patients with diabetes: a qualitative study. *Family Practice* 30, 113-118.
[60] Liu, X. N., Shinada, K., Chen, X. C., Zhang, B. X., Yaegaki, K. & Kawaguchi, Y. (2006) Oral malodor-related parameters in the Chinese general population. *Journal of Clinical Periodontology* 33, 31-36.
[61] Locker, D. (1988) Measuring oral health: a conceptual framework. *Community Dental Health* 5, 3-18.
[62] Locker, D. (1995) Health outcomes of oral disorders. *International Journal of Epidemiology* 24 Suppl 1, S85-89.
[63] Locker, D. (2004) Oral health and quality of life. *Oral Health and Preventive Dentistry* 2 Suppl 1, 247-253.
[64] Locker, D. & Allen, F. (2007) What do measures of 'oral health-related quality of life' measure? *Community Dentistry and Oral Epidemiology* 35, 401-411.
[65] Locker, D. & Miller, Y. (1994) Evaluation of subjective oral health status indicators. *Journal of Public Health Dentistry* 54, 167-176.
[66] Locker, D., Jokovic, A. & Clarke, M. (2004) Assessing the responsiveness of measures of oral health-related quality of life. *Community Dentistry and Oral Epidemiology* 32, 10-18.

[67] McGrath, C. & Bedi, R. (2001a) Can dental attendance improve quality of life? *British Dental Journal* 190, 262-265.

[68] McGrath, C. & Bedi, R. (2001b) An evaluation of a new measure of oral health related quality of life--OHQoL-UK(W). *Community Dental Health* 18, 138-143.

[69] McGrath, C. M., Bedi, R. & Gilthorpe, M. S. (2000) Oral health related quality of life--views of the public in the United Kingdom. *Community Dental Health* 17, 3-7.

[70] Misumi, S., Nakamoto, T., Kondo, Y., Mukaibo, T., Masaki, C. & Hosokawa, R. (2014) A prospective study of changes in oral health-related quality of life during immediate function implant procedures for edentulous individuals. *Clinical Oral Implants Research*, n/a-n/a.

[71] Mombelli, A., Cionca, N. & Almaghlouth, A. (2011) Does adjunctive antimicrobial therapy reduce the perceived need for periodontal surgery? *Periodontology 2000* 55, 205-216.

[72] Montero, J., Castillo-Oyague, R., Lynch, C. D., Albaladejo, A. & Castano, A. (2013) Self-perceived changes in oral health-related quality of life after receiving different types of conventional prosthetic treatments: a cohort follow-up study. *Journal of Dentistry* 41, 493-503.

[73] Needleman, I., McGrath, C., Floyd, P. & Biddle, A. (2004) Impact of oral health on the life quality of periodontal patients. *Journal of Clinical Periodontology* 31, 454-457.

[74] Ng, S. K. & Leung, W. K. (2006a) A community study on the relationship between stress, coping, affective dispositions and periodontal attachment loss. *Community Dentistry and Oral Epidemiology* 34, 252-266.

[75] Ng, S. K. & Leung, W. K. (2006b) Oral health-related quality of life and periodontal status. *Community Dentistry and Oral Epidemiology* 34, 114-122.

[76] Nikias, M. (1985) Oral disease and quality of life. *AmeriCan. J.ournal of Public Health* 75, 11-12.

[77] Oh, S. H., Kim, Y., Park, J. Y., Jung, Y. J., Kim, S. K. & Park, S. Y. (2014) Comparison of fixed implant-supported prostheses, removable implant-supported prostheses, and complete dentures: patient satisfaction and oral health-related quality of life. *Clinical Oral Implants Research*.

[78] Ozcelik, O., Haytac, M. C. & Seydaoglu, G. (2007) Immediate post-operative effects of different periodontal treatment modalities on oral health-related quality of life: a randomized clinical trial. *Journal of Clinical Periodontology* 34, 788-796.

[79] Paula, J. S., Leite, I. C., Almeida, A. B., Ambrosano, G. M., Pereira, A. C. & Mialhe, F. L. (2012) The influence of oral health conditions, socioeconomic status and home environment factors on schoolchildren's self-perception of quality of life. *Health and Quality of Life Outcomes* 10, 6.

[80] Pavel, K., Seydlova, M., Dostalova, T., Zdenek, V., Chleborad, K., Jana, Z., Feberova, J. & Radek, H. (2012) Dental implants and improvement of oral health-related quality of life. *Community Dentistry and Oral Epidemiology* 40 Suppl 1, 65-70.

[81] Petersen, P. E., Bourgeois, D., Ogawa, H., Estupinan-Day, S. & Ndiaye, C. (2005) The global burden of oral diseases and risks to oral health. *Bulletin of the World Health Organization* 83, 661-669.

[82] Pihlstrom, B. L., Hargreaves, K. M., Bouwsma, O. J., Myers, W. R., Goodale, M. B. & Doyle, M. J. (1999) Pain after periodontal scaling and root planing. *Journal of the American Dental Association* 130, 801-807.

[83] Rees, J. S., Jin, L. J., Lam, S., Kudanowska, I. & Vowles, R. (2003) The prevalence of dentine hypersensitivity in a hospital clinic population in Hong Kong. *Journal of Dentistry* 31, 453-461.

[84] Reisine, S. T. (1984) Dental Disease and Work Loss. *Journal of Dental Research* 63, 1158-1161.

[85] Richards, D. (2014) Review finds that severe periodontitis affects 11% of the world population. *Evidence-Based Dentistry* 15, 70-71.

[86] Ritz, L., Hefti, A. F. & Rateitschak, K. H. (1991) An *in vitro* investigation on the loss of root substance in scaling with various instruments. *Journal of Clinical Periodontology* 18, 643-647.

[87] Rousseau, N., Steele, J., May, C. & Exley, C. (2014) 'Your whole life is lived through your teeth': biographical disruption and experiences of tooth loss and replacement. *Sociology of Health and Illness* 36, 462-476.

[88] Saito, A., Hosaka, Y., Kikuchi, M., Akamatsu, M., Fukaya, C., Matsumoto, S., Ueshima, F., Hayakawa, H., Fujinami, K. & Nakagawa, T. (2010) Effect of initial periodontal therapy on oral health-related quality of life in patients with periodontitis in Japan. *Journal of Periodontology* 81, 1001-1009.

[89] Saito, A., Ota, K., Hosaka, Y., Akamatsu, M., Hayakawa, H., Fukaya, C., Ida, A., Fujinami, K., Sugito, H. & Nakagawa, T. (2011) Potential impact of surgical periodontal therapy on oral health-related quality of life in patients with periodontitis: a pilot study. *Journal of Clinical Periodontology* 38, 1115-1121.

[90] Sarita, P. T., Kreulen, C. M., Witter, D. & Creugers, N. H. (2003) Signs and symptoms associated with TMD in adults with shortened dental arches. *International Journal of Prosthodontics* 16, 265-270.

[91] Scully, C. & Greenman, J. (2008) Halitosis (breath odor). *Periodontology 2000* 48, 66-75.

[92] Shanbhag, S., Dahiya, M. & Croucher, R. (2012) The impact of periodontal therapy on oral health-related quality of life in adults: a systematic review. *Journal of Clinical Periodontology* 39, 725-735.

[93] Shugars, D. A., Benson, K., White, R. P., Jr., Simpson, K. N. & Bader, J. D. (1996) Developing a measure of patient perceptions of short-term outcomes of third molar surgery. *Journal of Oral and Maxillofacial Surgery* 54, 1402-1408.

[94] Simpson, T. C., Needleman, I., Wild, S. H., Moles, D. R. & Mills, E. J. (2010) Treatment of periodontal disease for glycaemic control in people with diabetes. *The Cochrane Database of Systematic Reviews*, CD004714.

[95] Slade, G. D. (1998) Assessing change in quality of life using the Oral Health Impact Profile. *Community Dentistry and Oral Epidemiology* 26, 52-61.

[96] Slade, G. D. & Spencer, A. J. (1994) Development and evaluation of the Oral Health Impact Profile. *Community Dental Health* 11, 3-11.

[97] Steele, J. G., Sanders, A. E., Slade, G. D., Allen, P. F., Lahti, S., Nuttall, N. & Spencer, A. J. (2004) How do age and tooth loss affect oral health impacts and quality of life? A study comparing two national samples. *Community Dentistry and Oral Epidemiology* 32, 107-114.

[98] Sukumar, S., John, M. T., Schierz, O., Aarabi, G. & Reissmann, D. R. (2015) Location of prosthodontic treatment and oral health-related quality of life - An exploratory study. *Journal of Prosthodontic Research* 59, 34-41.

[99] Suzuki, N., Yoneda, M., Naito, T., Iwamoto, T. & Hirofuji, T. (2008) Relationship between halitosis and psychologic status. *Oral Surgery, Oral Medicine, Oral Pathology, Oral Radiology and Endodontics* 106, 542-547.

[100] Tan, H., Peres, K. G. & Peres, M. A. (2014) Do people with shortened dental arches have worse oral health-related quality of life than those with more natural teeth? A population-based study. *Community Dentistry and Oral Epidemiology.*

[101] Tchicaya, A. & Lorentz, N. (2014) Socioeconomic inequalities in the non-use of dental care in Europe. *International Journal of Equity and Health* 13, 7.

[102] Thomason, J. M., Heydecke, G., Feine, J. S. & Ellis, J. S. (2007) How do patients perceive the benefit of reconstructive dentistry with regard to oral health-related quality of life and patient satisfaction? A systematic review. *Clinical Oral Implants Research* 18 Suppl 3, 168-188.

[103] Tobiasen, J. M. & Hiebert, J. M. (1993) Clefting and psychosocial adjustment. Influence of facial aesthetics. *Clinics in Plastic Surgery* 20, 623-631.

[104] Tomazoni, F., Zanatta, F. B., Tuchtenhagen, S., da Rosa, G. N., Del Fabro, J. P. & Ardenghi, T. M. (2014) Association of gingivitis with child oral health-related quality of life. *Journal of Periodontology* 85, 1557-1565.

[105] Tonetti, M. S., Fourmousis, I., Suvan, J., Cortellini, P., Bragger, U. & Lang, N. P. (2004) Healing, post-operative morbidity and patient perception of outcomes following regenerative therapy of deep intrabony defects. *Journal of Clinical Periodontology* 31, 1092-1098.

[106] Tonetti, M. S., Steffen, P., Muller-Campanile, V., Suvan, J. & Lang, N. P. (2000) Initial extractions and tooth loss during supportive care in a periodontal population seeking comprehensive care. *Journal of Clinical Periodontology* 27, 824-831.

[107] Tonetti, M. S. & Van Dyke, T. E. (2013) Periodontitis and atherosclerotic cardiovascular disease: consensus report of the Joint EFP/AAP Workshop on Periodontitis and Systemic Diseases. *Journal of Periodontology* 84, S24-29.

[108] Tsakos, G., Bernabe, E., D'Aiuto, F., Pikhart, H., Tonetti, M., Sheiham, A. & Donos, N. (2010) Assessing the minimally important difference in the oral impact on daily performances index in patients treated for periodontitis. *Journal of Clinical Periodontology* 37, 903-909.

[109] Tsakos, G., Gherunpong, S. & Sheiham, A. (2006) Can oral health-related quality of life measures substitute for normative needs assessments in 11 to 12-year-old children? *Journal of Public Health Dentistry* 66, 263-268.

[110] Vernazza, C., Heasman, P., Gaunt, F. & Pennington, M. (2012) How to measure the cost-effectiveness of periodontal treatments. *Periodontology 2000* 60, 138-146.

[111] von Troil, B., Needleman, I. & Sanz, M. (2002) A systematic review of the prevalence of root sensitivity following periodontal therapy. *Journal of Clinical Periodontology* 29 Suppl 3, 173-177; discussion 195-176.

[112] WHO (1948) Preamble to the Constitution of the World Health Organization as adopted by the International Health Conference, New York, 19-22 June, 1946; signed on 22 July 1946 by the representatives of 61 States (Official Records of the World Health Organization, no. 2, p. 100) and entered into force on 7 April 1948.

[113] WHO (1995) The World Health Organization Quality of Life assessment (WHOQOL): position paper from the World Health Organization. *Social Science and Medicine* 41, 1403-1409.

[114] Wilson, I. B. & Cleary, P. D. (1995) Linking clinical variables with health-related quality of life. A conceptual model of patient outcomes. *Journal of the American Medical Association* 273, 59-65.

[115] Witter, D. J., De Haan, A. F., Käyser, A. F. & Van Rossum, G. M. (1991) Shortened dental arches and periodontal support. *Journal of Oral Rehabilitation* 18, 203-212.

[116] Witter, D. J., De Haan, A. F., Käyser, A. F. & Van Rossum, G. M. (1994) A 6-year follow-up study of oral function in shortened dental arches. Part II: Craniomandibular dysfunction and oral comfort. *Journal of Oral Rehabilitation* 21, 353-366.

[117] Witter, D. J., van Elteren, P. & Käyser, A. F. (1987) Migration of teeth in shortened dental arches. *Journal of Oral Rehabilitation* 14, 321-329.

[118] Witter, D. J., Van Elteren, P., Käyser, A. F. & Van Rossum, G. M. (1990) Oral comfort in shortened dental arches. *Journal of Oral Rehabilitation* 17, 137-143.

[119] Witter, D. J., van Elteren, P., Käyser, A. F. & van Rossum, M. J. (1989) The effect of removable partial dentures on the oral function in shortened dental arches. *Journal of Oral Rehabilitation* 16, 27-33.

[120] Wong, R. M., Ng, S. K., Corbet, E. F. & Leung, W. K. (2012) Non-surgical periodontal therapy improves oral health-related quality of life. *Journal of Clinical Periodontology* 39, 53-61.

[121] Wood, P. H. (1980) The language of disablement: a glossary relating to disease and its consequences. *International Rehabilitation Medicine* 2, 86-92.

[122] Yach, D., Hawkes, C., Gould, C. L. & Hofman, K. J. (2004) The global burden of chronic diseases: overcoming impediments to prevention and control. *Journal of the American Medical Association* 291, 2616-2622.

[123] Yaegaki, K. & Coil, J. M. (2000) Examination, classification, and treatment of halitosis; clinical perspectives. *Journal of the Canadian Dental Association* 66, 257-261.

[124] Yu, S. J., Chen, P. & Zhu, G. X. (2013) Relationship between implantation of missing anterior teeth and oral health-related quality of life. *Quality of Life Research* 22, 1613-1620.

[125] Zaitsu, T., Ueno, M., Shinada, K., Wright, F. A. & Kawaguchi, Y. (2011) Social anxiety disorder in genuine halitosis patients. *Health and Quality of Life Outcomes* 9, 94.

[126] Zhang, Q., Witter, D. J., Gerritsen, A. E., Bronkhorst, E. M. & Creugers, N. H. (2013) Functional dental status and oral health-related quality of life in an over 40 years old Chinese population. *Clinical Oral Investigations* 17, 1471-1480.

In: Oral Health
Editor: Julia Renee Barnes

ISBN: 978-1-63482-832-1

Chapter II

Relationship between Periodontal Health and Its Impact on the Quality Life

A. L. Dumitrescu*
Bucharest, Romania

Abstract

Periodontal diseases are one of the common oral diseases involving structural and functional changes in the oral cavity and in their most severe forms are associated with formation of periodontal pockets, gingival abscesses, gingival recessions, tooth mobility, and finally teeth loss. Periodontal diseases are one of the main reasons for tooth loss among the population and this is furthermore related not only to alteration in speaking and chewing functions, but also to a high impact on the patients psychological and emotional well-being as related to daily social interactions, organ loss related trauma, self-esteem, shame, depression, anxiety. As a consequence, a better understanding of the consequences of periodontal disease is important in understanding patient perceptions of the impact of their gingival/periodontal health on their everyday lives, in planning periodontal therapy which addresses patient needs and in evaluating the results of the periodontal treatment from the patient's perspective. In the last decades, the relationship between individuals' periodontal health/therapy and quality of life has been extensively examined and this chapter reviews the current knowledge in this research field.

I. Introduction

Periodontal diseases are one of the common oral diseases involving structural and functional changes in the oral cavity and in their most severe forms are associated with

* Corresponding author: Email: E-mail: alexandrina_l_dumitrescu@yahoo.co.uk.

formation of periodontal pockets, gingival abscesses, gingival recessions, tooth mobility, and finally teeth loss (Figure 1). Periodontal diseases are one of the main reasons for tooth loss among the population and this is furthermore related not only to alteration in speaking and chewing functions, but also to a high impact on the patients psychological and emotional well-being as related to daily social interactions, organ loss related trauma, self-esteem, shame, depression, anxiety. As a consequence, a better understanding of the consequences of periodontal disease is important in understanding patient perceptions of the impact of their gingival/periodontal health on their everyday lives, in planning periodontal therapy which addresses patient needs and in evaluating the results of the periodontal treatment from the patient's perspective.

II. Oral Health-Related Quality of Life

II.1. Quality of Life - overview

Quality of life (QoL) is a concept difficult to define accurately, as the vast majority of definitions are centered on the notion of health as defined by the World Health Organization as "a state of complete, physical, mental and social well-being, and not merely the absence of disease or infirmity" (WHO, 1947; World Health Organization, 2005).

Quality of life (QoL) evaluations are providing clinicians with information regarding the general health of patients who might otherwise go unrecognized, thereby improving patient satisfaction and health outcomes. However, QoL measurements have not been routinely implemented in clinical practice and research, one concern expressed by clinicians being the questions about what QoL scales actually assess and how scores should be interpreted, especially as various diseases states (e.g., schizophrenia, Alzheimer's disease) and events (e.g., a stroke) may alter a person's perception of their physical and mental status, such as alterations in his metacognitive capabilities (metacognition defined as the ability to attribute mental states in terms of beliefs and goals to one's self and others) (Blanc et al., 2014). Self-reported QoL might be biased also by other psychological factors, such as adaptation to the illness. An important indicator of this adaptation process is an effect called the response shift, defined as changes in the meaning of one's self-evaluation of QoL resulting from changes in internal standards, values, or conceptualization (Sprangers and Schwartz, 1994a). Sprangers and Schwartz (1994a) proposed a theoretical model to clarify and predict changes in QoL as a result of the interaction of five major components: 1) a catalyst, 2) antecedents (e.g. sociodemographics (e.g. gender, education) and personality (e.g. optimism, self-esteem, sense of control, mastery), expectations or spiritual identity) , 3) mechanisms (e.g. using coping strategies, initiating social comparisons, seeking social support, reordering goals , reframing expectations and engaging in spiritual practice), 4) response shift and 5) perceived QoL (Sprangers and Schwartz, 1994a). The response shift refers to a change in the meaning of one's self-evaluation of a target construct as a result of: 1) recalibration defined as a change in the respondent's internal standards of scale measurement, 2) reprioritization defined as a change in the respondent's component domains constituting the target construct, QoL and 3) reconceptualization defined as a redefinition of QoL, the target construct (Figure 2) (Sprangers and Schwartz, 1994b). True changes of treatment effects may be over- or underestimated when an response shift is present, leading to biased estimates that are challenging mainly in interventional studies, in which patients' adaptation to treatment toxicities or disease progression over time side may change estimates of the true treatment effects (Sprangers and Schwartz, 1994b). Several protocols to assess response shift where described in aim to assess one or more of the three aspects of response shift (Sprangers and Schwartz, 1994b). Recently Vanier et al., (2015) suggested that the impact of the response shift effect on HRQL scores could be avoided (or lessened) if questionnaires were designed with a rule of "the least semantic and psychometric complexity" in mind.

In dental field, only a few studies have revealed the importance of taking into consideration the response shifts when evaluating the positive impact of dental treatment (Ring et al., 2005; Kimura et al., 2012; Reissmann et al., 2012) (Table 1).

Table 1. Impact of response shift on the assessment of dental treatment

Authors, year	**Study group**	**QoL instrument used**	**Conclusion**
Ring et al., 2005	117 patients (mean age 64.8; 32% male) evaluated at baseline (pre-test) and 3 months after receiving high quality conventional dentures (post-test).	Individualised quality of life (IQoL) measure, the SEIQoL	The positive impact of denture treatment for edentulous patients on IQoL was seen only when response shifts were taken into consideration.
Kimura et al., 2012	73 consecutive patients with no more than eight missing teeth who received implant-supported, fixed or removable partial dentures were asked to complete the full-version OHRQoL questionnaire before (pre-test) and after treatment (post-test) (1 year later).	Oral Health-Related Quality of Life (OHRQoL)	The significant predictor variables for the response shift were young age, fewer numbers of replaced teeth and lower pre-test scores.
Reissmann et al., 2012	A consecutive sample of 126 patients seeking prosthodontic care. Patients were asked to rate their OHRQoL before treatment started and 1 month after treatment was finished.	Oral Health Impact Profile (OHIP)	The response shift phenomenon and its magnitude have important implications for dental practice, where patients and dentists often assess perceived treatment effects retrospectively

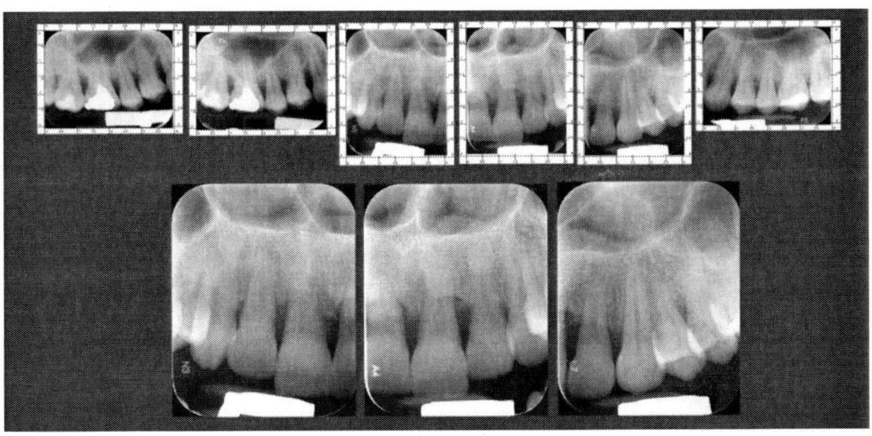

Figure 1. Radiograph showing advanced bone loss in moderate to severe periodontal disease

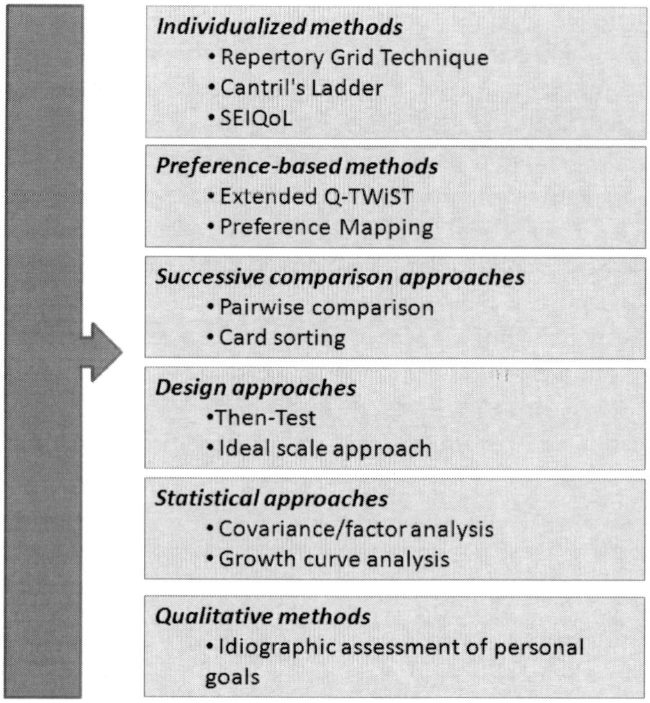

Figure 2. Methods for assessing response shift (Sprangers and Schwartz, 1994b).

II.2. Health-Related Quality of Life (HRQoL) - Overview

The term "Health-related Quality of Life" (HRQoL) is a concept frequently used in aim to highlight on the relationship between health and quality of life. According to the Ferrans Conceptual Model HRQoL includes four domains areas related to physical, mental and emotional, and social functioning (Ferrans, 2005). HRQoL goes beyond the direct measures of health and focuses on the quality-of-life consequences of health status, playing a crucial role in clinical decision-making care, through its contribution to targeting of problems, identification of the balance between positive and negative effects of therapy, identification of the need for supportive care and improvement of physician-patient communication (Halyard and Ferrans, 2008). Moreover, several regulatory agencies (e.g. International Society for Quality of Life Research, Global Allergy and Asthma European Network (GA2LEN), National Cancer Institute, American Society of Clinical oncology, Canadian Cardiovascular Society) recommend assessing quality of life (QoL) in daily clinical practice in patients with chronic illnesses (Aaronson et al., 2011; Baiardini et al., 2010; Halyard and Ferrans, 2008; Bower et al., 2014; Boodhwani et al., 2014).

An important aspect is that, from the perspective of patients, QoL and health status are distinct constructs and the two terms should not be used interchangeably. When rating QoL, patients give greater emphasis to mental health than to physical functioning. However, this model is inverted for appraisals of health status, for which mental health is less important than physical functioning. Social functioning did not have a major impact on either construct. These facts have a relevant research consequence as many important health status scales, including utility-based questionnaires and health perception indexes, may be inappropriate for measuring QoL, while evaluations of the effectiveness of medical treatment may differ depending on whether QoL or health status is the study outcome (Smith et al., 1999).

HRQoL include several core concepts:

- **subjectively**: includes the need of a subjective input from the affected person regarding both positive and negative responses to illness and treatment (Cella and Nowinski, 2002);
- **multidimensionality**: a full appreciation of the impact of illness and treatment requires assessment of a broad spectrum of functioning and well-being, such as symptoms, physical functioning, mood, cognition, family functioning, and social activity (Cella and Nowinski, 2002);
- **dynamism**: can change over time as individual attitudes are not constant, vary with time and experience, and are modified by psychological factors such as coping, expectancy, optimism and adaptation (Allison et al., 1997).

There are many **HRQoL models** applied across different health and illness conditions, across the lifespan,and among individuals, their families, and communities as recently reviewed (Bakas et al., 2012; Costa and King, 2013). Three HRQoL disease-specific models models were selected by the systematic review performed by Bakas et al., (2012):

- Wilson and Cleary's (1995) model of HRQoL combines two paradigms, biomedical and social science and includes five major well-defined domains: biological, symptoms, function, general health perception, and overall HRQoL that are inter-related with reciprocal relationships;
- Ferrans et al., (2005) model retained the five major domains of the Wilson and Cleary's (1995) HRQoL model, but was also revised in three substantive ways: a) indicating that biological function is influenced by characteristics of both individuals and environments; b) deleting nonmedical factors; and c) deleting the labels on the arrows that tend to restrict characterization of the relationships. In addition, they provided examples of of instruments to measure the major components of the model (Ferrans and Powers, 1995). The revised Ferrans et al., (2005) model can be applied to any health care discipline;
- The World Health Organization International Classification of Functioning, Disability, and Health (WHO ICF) (World Health Organization, 1980; World Health Organization, 2001; World Health Organization, 2007) is a model that covers various age groups (from children and adolescents to adults) and provides a unified and standard description of health and health states that can be used across disciplines and cultures. The WHO ICF model includes components within two main parts: 1) main functioning and disability (body functioning and structures, activities, and participation), and 2) Contextual factors (environmental and personal). However, the WHO ICF is not specific to the area of HRQoL but rather represents a mapping and classification framework.

HRQoL assessments are divided into two general types (Patrick and Deyo, 1989; Cella and Nowinski, 2002):

- **Disease-specific assessments** are targeted for patients with a specific condition or treatment under study and, as a result, tend to be more responsive to clinically important changes than generic instruments. The disadvantages of the targeted-instruments are: 1) they may lack items pertaining to dimensions of the disease that affects QoL, and thus are not accurately reflect patient's QoL; 2) are not easy to be used for the comparisons of different populations or different interventions (Patrick and Deyo, 1989; Cella and Nowinski, 2002). Examples of specific instruments are: Parkinson's Disease Questionnaire (Marinus et al., 2002), McGill's quality of life questionnaire (used for persons with life-threatening illnesses)(De Maeyer et al., 2010), Lancashire QoL profile (used for persons with mental health problems)(van Nieuwenhuizen et al., 2001) or Inflammatory Bowel Disease Questionnaire (Irvine, 1993).
- **Generic assessments** have the advantage to allow for broad evaluation of overall health across many different domains, to offer the possibility to compare results across different groups of patients, population cohorts and interventions, and some can provide normative or benchmark data from which to interpret results. The disadvantages of the generic assessments are the involuntarily bias results toward or against subsets of the general population (Patrick and Deyo, 1989; Cella and Nowinski, 2002).

Generic instruments can be divided into single instruments and health profiles:

- Single global health measures (e.g. "How do you rate your health status") have been shown to be reliable and valid and have been recommended for use in health monitoring by the US Centres for Disease Control, the WHO, the European Commission (Salomon et al., 2009; Hennessy et al., 1994) and in the American public health plan Healthy People 2010 (Andresen et al., 2003).
- Health profiles are instruments "that attempt to measure all important aspects of HRQoL" (Guyatt et al., 1993). Several papers described (Cella and Nowinski, 2002; Patrick and Deyo, 1989; Ferrans, 2005; Halyard and Ferrans, 2008; Allison et al., 1997; Aaronson et al., 1993; Cella et al., 1997; Wu et al., 2001; Cella et al., 2007; Haywood et al., 2005; Cagney et al., 2000) or summarized (Haywood et al., 2006; Haywood et al., 2005a; Haywood et al., 2005b) the most common HRQoL instruments: Dartmouth COOP Charts for Primary Care Practice, WONCA/COOP, Functional Status Questionnaire/FSQ, Goteborg Quality of Life/GQL, Health Status Questionnaire-12/HSQ-12, Nottingham Health Profile/NHP, Quality of Life Index/QLI, Quality of Well-being - Self-administered/QWB-SA, Short Form 12-item Health Survey/SF-12, Short Form 20-item Health Survey/SF-20, Short Form 36-item Health Survey/SF-36, Sickness Impact Profile/SIP, Spitzer Quality of Life, The sickness impact profile (SIP), World Health Organization Quality of Life (WHOQoL Bref), EuroQoL-5D (EQ-5D) and SF-36.

When choosing a HRQoL assessment tool it is important to comprehend the background and patient population in which the instrument was designed, because this affects the reliability and validity of the expected QoL (Patrick and Deyo, 1989). Because no single instrument is ideal in all situations, researchers and clinicians prefer to use **a mixture of**

generic and disease-specific scales (e.g. a core generic instrument to assess the common HRQoL dimensions associated with several targeted subscales specific to the disease, condition, or intervention of interest) in aim to benefit from on the strengths of both, while minimizing the limitations of each. For longitudinal use, the serial assessment of HRQoL may be a helpful method to scrutinize disease course and response to therapy (Cella and Nowinski, 2002).

II.3. Oral Health-Related Quality of Life - Overview

As Locker mentioned since 1997: "from the point of view of contemporary definitions of health, epidemiological measures in terms of DMFT [decayed missing filled teeth] and CPITN [community periodontal index of treatment needs] have serious limitations in that they tell us nothing about the functioning of the oral cavity or the person as a whole and nothing about subjectively perceived symptoms such as pain and discomfort."

Most oral diseases (e.g. dental caries, periodontal diseases) may cause pain and suffering, and have physical, economical, social, and psychological consequences that can have a critically effect on a range of aspects of life, such as appearance, oral function, and interpersonal relationships, which ultimately prejudice the quality of life in both adults and children (Gilbert et al., 1998; Gomes and Abegg, 2007; Masood et al., 2014). For example, parents or guardians of 4-yrs children with severe caries revealed that oral health affects their children's life: the children complained of toothache, had problems eating certain foods, were absent from school, were ashamed to smile, and stopped playing with other children because of their teeth (Feitosa et al., 2005).

Oral Health-related Quality of Life (OHRQoL) is an emerging subject of importance during recent years and has been defined as a **subset of Health-related Quality of Life** (McGrath and Bedi, 2002; John et al., 2003). OHRQoL **is multidimensional** and is closely related to socio-demographic characteristics (e.g. age, gender, ethnicity), economic (e.g. household income) and cultural aspects (McGrath and Bedi, 2002; Sisson, 2007). Moreover, individuals with lower socioeconomic status are exposed to material deprivation which could influence their engaging in riskier behaviors, resulting in more severe impacts on their OHRQoL (Peres et al., 2007). Similar with HRQoL, OHRQoL is also **dynamic** over time and practice (Allison et al., 1997). For example, untreated /complicated caries may lead to eating problems, but when oral cancer has been diagnosed, the same person may have more problems when eating, but they become less important comparing with the main diagnosis (Allison et al., 1997). Several **models of oral health and OHRQoL** have been reviewed by Brondani and MacEntee, (2014) and as most models are based on negative biomedical view of oral disorders and do not willingly accommodate the biopsychosocial theories of oral health, alternative emerged models showed a change in the understanding of oral health beyond illness and included dynamically positive behaviours and adaptive strategies (Williams et al., 1998; MacEntee, 2006).

However, there are large differences in the total number of studies on HRQoL and OHRQoL, as the number of entries on PubMed with HRQoL and OHRQoL was on 6th March 2015 44 823 publications (6 699 reviews), respectively 2 719 publications (399 reviews). According to the ICI web of knowledge, at the same time, the number of papers related to the HRQoL was 44 284 while for OHRQoL was 2 353.

Measurements of oral health and OHRQoL have been designed in a similar way as HRQoL scales (Inglehart, 2006; John, 2007):

A) **Generic assessments** were divided into single question and multi-item instruments.

- **Single global health measures** (e.g. "How do you rate your oral health status?"): Pattussi et al., (2007) described this question as a simple and easy way to collect dental health information, while Locker and Jokovic (2007) mentioned "that these single item measures provide a summary of how people perceive their health, both objective and subjective, and that they may be as useful as more complex multi-item scales and indexes in health status assessments." However, "despite its use in medical studies, a single question of self rated oral health has seldom been used as the primary outcome in dental studies" even it is "an economical way of summarizing the state of a person's oral health" (Dolan et al., 1998). This short one-item instrument is also usually used as gold standard in validity studies of multi-item scales (Agou et al., 2008;Allen et al., 2009; Baker, 2007; Jokovic et al., 2004; Jokovic et al., 2004; Jones et al., 2004; Li et al., 2008; Locker et al., 2004; Locker 2008; Pahel et al., 2007; Bernabe et al., 2008; Castro et al., 2008; Ostberg et al., 2001). Moreover, the clinical validity of Locker's global self-reported oral health item as a global self-reported oral health measure in young middle-aged adults was recently demonstrated by Thomson et al., (2012). In a similar way, the Oral Satisfaction Scale (OSS) was designed as a visual analogue scale (0 to 10) that allows participants to evaluate their perceived oral satisfaction, representing a measure of psychological well-being in relation with mouth (Montero et al., 2008).
- **The multi-item inventories** are also called socio-dental indicators (SDIs) and were used mainly in cross-sectional studies for psychometric evaluation and investigation of prevalence of oral impacts in different populations (Slade et al., 1996; Baker et al., 2006; Atchison and Dolan, 1990; Åstrøm and Okullo, 2003; Gilchrist et al., 2014). These SDIs emphasize a range of behavioural and functional disturbances triggerend from the dental area that affect the lives of people from all age groups (Slade 1997). A high number of SDIs have been developed in the last 30 years and were summarized in different studies (Slade, 1997; Jones et al., 2004; Bourgeois and Lodra 2004; Hebling and Pereira 2007; Brondani and MacEntee, 2007; Locker and Allen, 2007; Riordain and McCreary, 2010). Among these multi-item inventories can be mentioned: the Social Impacts of Dental Disease (SIDD), the Rand Dental questionnaire, the Geriatric Oral Health Assessment Index (GOHAI), the Oral Health-related Quality of Life Measure (OHQoL), the Dental Impact Profile (DIP), the Oral Health Impact Profile (OHIP), as well many others presented in **Table 2.** Several of these questionnaires were designed to assess the OHRQoL specifically in children: Child Perception Questionnaire (CPQ $_{11\text{-}14}$), the Michigan OHRQoL scale, the Child Oral Health Impact Profile (Child-OHIP), the Early Childhood Oral Health Impact Scale (ECOHIS), Child Oral Impact on Daily Performance (Child-OIDP), Scale of Oral Health Outcomes for 5-year-old children (SOHO-5), Child Oral Health-Related Quality of Life for 8-10-year-olds (COHRQoL [8-10]) and the Oral Health related Early Childhood Quality of Life (OH- ECQOL) scale.

Table 2. Examples of currently available OHQoL measures

Instrument	Abbreviation	No. of items	Original reference
Child Oral Health Impact Profile	COHIP	34	Broder, 2007
Child Oral Health Impact Profile-Short Form 19	COHIP-SF 19	19	Broder et al., 2012
Child Oral Health Quality of Life questionnaire consists of 1) Child Perception Questionnaire, 2) Parental Perception Questionnaire, and 3) Family Impact Scale	COHQoL 1)CPQ11–14 2)PPQ 3)FIS	 36 31 14	Jokovic et al., 2002a, Jokovic et al., 2002b, Jokovic et al., 2003, Jokovic et al., 2004
Child Oral Health-Related Quality of Life for 8-10-year-olds	COHRQoL (8-10)	25	Humphris et al., 2005
Child-Oral Impacts on Daily Performances	CHILD-OIDP	8	Gherunpong et al., 2004
DENTAL	DENTAL	15	Bush et al., 1996
Dental Impact on Daily Living	DIDL	36	Leao and Sheiham, 1996
Dental Impact Profile	DIP	25	Strauss and Hunt, 1993
Early childhood oral health impact scale	ECOHIS	13	Pahel et al., 2007
Family Impact Scale	FIS	14	Locker and Allen, 2002
Geriatric (General) Oral Health Assessment Index	GOHAI	12	Atchison and Dolan, 1990
OHQoL-UK(W)		16	McGrath and Bedi, 2001
OHRQOL for Dental Hygiene		56	Gadbdury-Amyot et al., 1999
OHRQoL measure	OHRQoL	3	Kressin et al., 1996
Oral Health Impact Profile	OHIP-49	49	Slade and Spencer, 1994
Oral Health Impact Profile	OHIP-14	14	Slade, 1997
Oral Health Impact Profile (OHIP-EDENT)	OHIP-20	20	Allen and Locker, 2002
Oral Health Index	OHS	3	Burke et al., 2003
Oral Health Quality of life – UK (United Kingdom)	OHRQoL-UK	16	McGrath and Bedi, 2001
Oral Health Quality of Life Inventory	OHQol	15	Cornell et al., 1997
Oral Health related Early Childhood Quality of Life	OH-ECQOL	16	Mathur et al., 2014
Oral Health-related Quality of Life Measure from the Rand Health Insurance Study (Rand Dental Health Index)	OHQoL	3	Dolan et al., 1991

Table 2. (Continued)

Instrument	Abbreviation	No. of items	Original reference
Oral Impact on Daily Performances	OIDP	8	Adulyanon and Sheiham, 1997
Oral Impacts on Daily Performances index	OIDP	8	Montero et al., 2008
Orthognathic Quality of Life Questionnaire	OQoLQ	22	Cunningham et al., 2000
Psychosocial impact score		42	Locker and Miller, 1994
Scale of Oral Health Outcomes for 5-year-old children	SOHO-5	7	Tsakos et al., 2012
Sickness Impact Profile	SIP	73	Bergner et al., 1981
Social Impact of Dental Disease	SIDD	14	Cushing et al., 1986
Subjective Oral Health Status Indicators (index of chewing capacity, index of the ability to speak clearly, index of oral and facial pain symptoms, index of other oral symptoms.)	SOHSI	28	Locker and Miller, 1994
Surgical Orthodontic Outcome Questionnaire	SOOQ	33	Locker et al., 2007
The DELTA		6	Jones et al., 2003

Table 3. Summary of studies evaluating the impact of gingival health status on OHQoL. Review of studies during the period 2000–2015

Author/year	Country	Study group /age	Gingival evaluation	OHQoL instrument used	Study result
Tomazoni et al., 2014	Brazil	1,134 schoolchildren / 12-year- old	Community Periodontal Index	Child Perceptions Questionnaire for 11- to 14-Year-Old Children (CPQ11-14)	The presence of extensive levels of gingivitis might be negatively associated with how children perceive their oral health and their daily life.
Amato et al., 2014	Brazil	50 students / 11-12 year old	Community Periodontal Index and two questions about gingival bleeding	Child Oral Impacts on Daily Performances (Child-OIDP)	A significant improvement in the clinical status and oral hygiene was associated with a significant decline in the Child-OIDP scores.

Author/year	Country	Study group /age	Gingival evaluation	OHQoL instrument used	Study result
Nanayakkara et al., 2013	Sri Lanka	784 children aged between 48-72 months	Bleeding Index	Early Childhood Oral Health Impact Scale (ECOHIS)	Children with more gingival bleeding (bleeding surfaces) presented a poorer OHQoL
Cornejo et al., 2013	Argentina	Eighty pregnant women/ age 18-39 yrs	Gingival Index (Löe and Silness, 1963); depth on probing, clinical attachment level, bleeding on probing	OHIP-49	Oral health status and oral health-related quality of life showed no significant association.
Krisdapong al., 2012b	Thailand	1,100 children 12-year-old	Community Periodontal Index (CPI)	Child-Oral Impacts on Daily Performances (Child-OIDP)	Children with gingivitis or calculus in three or more sextants were twice as likely and children with calculus and gingivitis in three or more sextants were 3.5 times more likely to report condition-specific impacts.
Zanatta et al., 2012	Brazil	330 participants under fixed orthodontic treatment	Bleeding on probing (BOP), PD, CAL, gingival enlargement	Oral Health Impact Profile (OHIP-14)	Anterior gingival enlargement seems to influence the OHRQoL in subjects receiving orthodontic treatment.
Krisdapong et al., 2012c	Thailand	871 adolescents 15-year-old	Community Periodontal Index (CPI)	Oral Impacts on Daily Performances (OIDP)	Adolescents with extensive gingivitis in 3 or more mouth sextants were twice as likely to experience moderate/higher condition-specific impacts
Krisdapong et al., 2012d	Thailand	1,063 twelve-year olds and 811 fifteen-year olds	Community Periodontal Index (CPI)	Child-Oral Impacts on Daily Performances (Child-OIDP) and Oral Impacts on Daily Performances (OIDP)	Gingivitis was generally associated with any level of condition-specific-impacts attributed to calculus and/or gingivitis. Condition-specific impacts were related more to gingivitis than to calculus.

Table 3. (Continued)

Author/year	Country	Study group /age	Gingival evaluation	OHQoL instrument used	Study result
Barbosa et al., 2009	Brazil	210 children aged 8–14 years	Community Periodontal Index (CPI)	Child Perceptions Questionnaires (CPQ8-10 and CPQ11-14)	Children without gingivitis had $CPQ_{8–10}$ higher scores for the overall and emotional well-being domains.
Acharya et al., 2009	India	259 pregnant women (mean age 26 +/- 5.5 yrs)	Gingival index, Community Periodontal Index of Treatment Needs (CPITN)	Oral Health Impact Profile (OHIP-14)	Gingival index scores, community periodontal index of treatment needs scores and previous pregnancies were associated with poorer OHRQoL scores.
Acharya, 2008	India	414 general dental patients	Gingival index	Oral Health Impact Profile (OHIP-14), General health questionnaire (GHQ)-12	The results of this study showed that caries status, psychological distress and dental anxiety had an important effect on the OHRQoL
López and Baelum, 2007	Chile	9203 high school students	Clinical attachment level, The presence of necrotizing ulcerative gingivitis	Oral Health Impact Profile (OHIP-14)	Both attachment loss [OR = 2.0] and necrotizing ulcerative gingivitis [OR = 1.6] were significantly associated with higher impact on the Oral Health Related Quality of Life of adolescents.
Robinson et al., 2005	Ugand	174 children 12 year old	Community Periodontal Index (CPI)	Child Oral Health Related Quality of Life (CPQ11-14)	The number of sites with gingivitis or the presence of calculus or trauma were not associated with summary measures of CPQ11-14 whereas having any dental caries or treatment experience was associated with higher total scores and more impacts.

Author/year	Country	Study group /age	Gingival evaluation	OHQoL instrument used	Study result
Marshman et al., 2005	UK	89 children between 11 and 14 years	Community Periodontal Index (CPI)	Child Perceptions Questionnaire (CPQ11-14)	Number of impacts correlated with the total number of missing teeth and missing teeth due to caries. No other relationships between clinical and CPQ11-14 data were apparent
Needleman et al., 2004	UK	205 patients attending a private periodontal clinic	Check list of questions about their periodontal health over the past year	UK oral health-related quality-of-life measure (OHQoL-UK)	OHQoL-UK scores were associated with patient's self-reported periodontal health in the past year: experiences of "swollen gums," "sore gums," "receding gums," "loose teeth,” "drifting teeth," "bad breath" and "toothache"

B) **Specific impacts measures**, designed for evaluation of pain, taste, impaired speech or appearance are also commonly used in cited in oral health surveys (Reisine et al., 1989; Gilbert et al., 1993; Krisdapong et al., 2012). Moreover, it was revealed that condition-specific instruments have better discriminative ability than generic OHRQoL scales (Bernabe et al., 2008; Bernabe et al., 2009). Several specific OHQoL impacts scales have been designed:

- FACE-Q Oncology is a new patient-reported outcome instrument for HRQoL evaluation following head and neck cancer reconstruction (Albornoz et al., 2013);
- Quality of Life with Implant-Prostheses' (QoLIP-10) questionnaire was developed for assessing the OHRQoL of implant-prosthesis wearers (Preciado et al., 2013);
- Pain-related limitations of daily function in the TMD questionnaire (LDF-TMDQ, 13 items) scale has been designed to assess oral health-related quality of life in patients with temporomandibular disorders (TMDs) (Sugisaki et al., 2005);
- The Liverpool Oral Rehabilitation Questionnaire (LORQ) was designed to record patient-derived outcomes in head and neck cancer. The questionnaire consists of 25 items about oral function and denture satisfaction (Pace-Balzan et al., 2004);
- The Scale Assessing the Impact of Periodontal Diseases on Patients' Quality of Life (Musurlieva et al., 2012) contains 9 items grouped in three subscales that assess a) the patient's choice of food/nutrition, chewing, swallowing, b) social relations, friends and family, professional and c) overall health. The scale presented a Cronbach's α coefficient = 0.883 and an average inter-item correlation coefficient 0.507.

III. Impact of Gingival Inflammation/Gingivitis on Oral Health-Related Quality of Life

Gingival aspect is one of the components of the smile's harmony. The smile not only is used to express different feelings (e.g. joy, success, kindness, sensuality, affection), but, more important, represents one of the most important physical characteristics involved in the self-esteem, self-confidence and self-image. People dissatisfied with their own smile are most commonly affected with an unpleasant appearance, are less self-confident, to have a lower self-esteem and to like themselves less than those who are satisfied (Albashaireh et al., 2009; Van der Geld et al., 2007; Pinho et al., 2007).

Evidence shows that gingival bleeding and enlargement is associated not only with aesthetic problems, phonetic alterations and masticatory problems, but also with alterations in OHQoL (**Table 3.**).

Self-reported gingival bleeding, one of the main clinical signs of gingivitis, was associated with higher self-focused attention (Dumitrescu et al., 2011a), body-related shame (Dumitrescu et al., 2011b), higher values of dental anxiety and lower levels of self-esteem (Dumitrescu et al., 2010), lower values of self-liking, self-competence and body investment

(Dumitrescu et al., 2009a), lower levels of self-confidence and of self-control (Dumitrescu et al., 2009b), higher values of social anxiety (Dumitrescu et al., 2008a), lower body appreciation (Dumitrescu et al., 2008b), reduced social desirability (Dumitrescu et al., 2007a), and higher perceived stress (Dumitrescu et al., 2007b).

Moreover, it was showed that self-reported gingival bleeding was associated among undergraduate students with statistical significant higher values of self-blame and rumination, while participants who evaluated their self-reported gingival condition as poor/very poor scored higher values on rumination, catastrophising and lower on positive reappraisal, when compared with students with excellent gingival condition (Dumitrescu et al., 20011c).

IV. Impact of Periodontal Health on Oral Health-Related Quality of Life

Periodontal diseases are one of the common oral diseases involving structural and functional changes in the oral cavity and in their most severe forms are associated with formation of periodontal pockets, gingival abscesses, gingival recessions, tooth mobility, and finally teeth loss. Periodontal diseases are one of the main reasons for tooth loss among the population and this is furthermore related not only to alteration in speaking and chewing functions, but also to a high impact on the patients psychological and emotional well-being as related to daily social interactions, organ loss related trauma, self-esteem, shame, depression, anxiety. As a consequence, a better understanding of the consequences of periodontal disease is important in understanding patient perceptions of the impact of their gingival/periodontal health on their everyday lives, in planning periodontal therapy which addresses patient needs and in evaluating the results of the periodontal treatment from the patient's perspective.

In dental studies, periodontal disease is usually evaluated by therapist-centered surrogate endpoints such as bleeding on probing (BOP), probing depth PD and clinical attachment level (CAL) (Slade et al., 1998), but rarely by patient-centered measures. However, a recent number of studies have investigated and have demonstrated that periodontal disease does have a negative impact on patients' oral health quality of life due to mastication, nutritional problems, physical pain and psychological disability (Gil-Montoya et al., 2015; DeBaz et al., 2015; Gil-Montoya et al., 2015; Jansson et al., 2014; Brauchle et al., 2013; Sundaram et al., 2013; Eltas A, Uslu 2013; Durham et al., 2013; Cornejo et al., 2013; Nagarajan et al., 2012; Al Habashneh et al., 2012; Musurlieva et al., 2012; Zaitsu et al., 2011; Li et al., 2011; Tsakos et al., 2010; Araújo et al., 2010; O'Dowd et al., 2010; Jowett et al., 2009; Cunha-Cruz et al., 2007; Barer et al., 2007; Ng SK, Leung WK. 2006; Needleman et al., 2004; Karlsson et al., 2009; Brennan et al., 2007 ; Lawrence et al., 2008 ; Mariño et al., 2008 ; Durham et al., 2013), also reveled by a recent systematic review (Al-Harthi et al., 2013). It has been reported also a correlation between extent and/or severity of periodontal disease and poorer OHRQoL, the strength of the association being reported to be either an OR of 1.5 (95% CI = 1.02–2.19) to 2.0 (95% CI = 1.5–2.5), or RR = 1.3 (95% CI = 1.2–1.4) (Al-Harthi et al., 2013; Needleman et al., 2004; Ng & Leung 2006; Cunha-Cruz et al., 2007; Bernabe & Marcenes, 2010).

It was also revealed that, when the patients with periodontal disease faced the fact that it was not possible to keep the teeth any longer, followed a period of fear, shame and denial, with a direct negative effect on their social life (Johannsen et al., 2012). A qualitative study that investigated patients' perceptions of living with periodontitis identified two main categories: first, the patients' perception of what causes periodontitis, being given the diagnosis, after the diagnosis and the consequences of periodontitis, and the second category reveals the patients' perception of their own responsibility and the professionals' responsibility (Karlsson et al., 2009). The authors suggested that acceptance and control of the disease may cause less difficulties in the patients' daily lives and may lead to a more positive future perspective, despite feelings of anxiety about long-term consequences such as edentations due to tooth loss (Karlsson et al., 2009).

Patient-based outcomes (PBOs) or "true endpoints" such as OHQoL were also investigated in periodontal therapy as patients' opinions may differ from traditional clinical endpoints (Aslund et al., 2008; Brauchle et al., 2013; Del Fabbro et al., 2009; Franke et al., 2014; Jönsson and Öhrn 2014; Nagarajan and Chandra 2012; Ozcelik et al., 2007; Jowett et al., 2009; Saito et al., 2010; Saito et al., 2011; Sundaram et al., 2013; Wong et al., 2012; Shanbhag et al., 2012). A recent systematic review summarized these studies and revealed that all forms of non-surgical periodontal therapy can improve the OHRQoL of adult patients with periodontal disease in the immediate (1 week) and long-term (12 months) (Shanbhag et al., 2012), in the domains of function, psychology and pain. In contrast, when provided alone surgical periodontal treatment may be associated with more negative impacts and when performed in patients who have already received non-surgical periodontal therapy does not have a significant additional benefit on the OHRQoL (Shanbhag et al., 2012).

V. Impact of Edentulism on Oral Health-Related Quality of Life

Periodontal disease is a chronic, destructive condition characterized gums inflammation and the gradual destruction of periodontal tissues and alveolar bone supporting the teeth. As a consequence, periodontitis, a disease that affects a large number of the adult population, is one of the major causes of tooth loss in adults (Papapanou, 1996; Irfan et al., 2001).

A recent systematic review provided fairly strong evidence that tooth loss impair OHRQoL (Gerritsen et al., 2010). Tooth loss has an impact of on the quality of life through both a physical (e.g. difficulties in eating) and social dimensions (e.g. problems in communication with other people)(Saintrain and de Souza, 2012; Nguyen et al., 2011; Visscher et al., 2014; Huang and Park, 2014; Dable et al., 2014; Gülcan et al., 2014; Batista et al., 2014; Zhang et al., 2013; Pistorius et al., 2013; Singh and Brennan, 2012; Saintrain and de Souza, 2012).

This association is independent from the OHRQoL instrument used and context (e.g., cultural background), but the extent and severity of impairment seems to be **context dependent.** The prevalence of negative impacts increases sharply once the number of teeth present drops below 20 (Gerritsen et al., 2010). Otherwise, the quantity of teeth lost does not affect OHRQoL, but rather should be taken in consideration the number of occluding pairs, location and distribution of missing teeth (Gerritsen et al., 2010; Batista et al., 2014; Somsak and Kaewplung, 2014).

Among older people, long-term routine attendance had positive impact on major tooth loss and OHRQoL supporting the principle of encouraging annual dental attendance for preventive checkups (Åstrøm et al., 2014).

However, the studies under analysis were mainly population based and not **individual based**. Rousseau et al., (2014) revealed that while for some individuals the loss of a tooth is relatively insignificant, for others it is devastating and disruptive. Two forms of biographical disruption were identified: the first was connected to the meanings of tooth loss (the neglected mouth) and denture wearing (a marker of old age), while the second disruption was embodied and was linked to the relationship between the self and mouth in those wearing dentures (the invaded, unreliable mouth) and could take place even where tooth loss and denture wearing had been biographically anticipated (Rousseau et al., 2014). When the influence of **personality traits** was investigated, negative affectivity was statistically and clinically significantly higher and self-esteem was statistically significantly lower in patients reporting worse oral comfort and OHRQoL (Özhayat, 2013). Preservation of teeth had a positive effect on QoL as it contributes to a positive body image, self-worth, pride and achievement, intactness, and sense of control (Niesten et al., 2012), and to a reduced vulnerability (De Marchi et al., 2012). There seems to be a gender effect in that the men generally care less about having natural teeth than women (Niesten et al., 2012).

The influence of the replacement of tooth loss on OHQoL was also investigated:

- One systematic review performed by Hultin et al., (2012) revealed that the oral rehabilitation following total or partial tooth loss has positive influence on self-perceived OHRQoL.
- When the cost-effectiveness of conventional treatment using partial dentures with functionally orientated treatment to replace missing teeth for partially dentate elders was compared, it was reported an improvements in OHRQoL 1 month after completion of treatment either through conventional (e.g. removable partial dentures to replace all missing natural teeth) or functionally orientated therapy (e.g. Shortened Dental Arch (SDA) restoration of 10 occluding contacts using resin-bonded bridgework)(McKenna et al., 2013).
- In completely edentulous patients, over 65 yrs of age, there was a significant change in the quality of life in elderly after their prosthodontic rehabilitation, though the self rated general health did not show any significant improvement (Dable et al., 2013) with a higher increase of patient satisfaction and OHQoL in the mandibular implant-retained overdenture compared to conventional dentures (Emami et al., 2013), especially when frontal teeth are affected (Yu et al., 2013).
- In edentulous patients, the treatment with dental implants increased OHQoL, improved function, self-esteem and social life (Johannsen et al., 2012);
- The evaluation of the OHQoL in a population about to receive removable dental prostheses or fixed dental prostheses revealed that the most frequently reported problems in all groups concerned functional limitations, discomfort and physical disabilities. Higher age was significantly correlated with a better OHRQoL independent of treatment modality. However, patients who received fixed dental prostheses in one jaw in the masticatory zone only had a better OHRQoL than participants who received removable dental prostheses in the same group (Özhayat and Gotfredsen, 2013).

Conclusion

As far as we can see, periodontal disease has a tremendous impact on the patients' quality of life, in all of her dimensions, and it is the responsibility of the entire dental community to understand the psychological needs of their patients under the dental care.

References

[1] Aaronson, NK; Ahmedzai, S; Bergman, B; Bullinger, M; Cull, A; Duez, NJ; Filiberti, A; Flechtner, H; Fleishman, SB; de Haes, JC; et al., The European Organization for Research and Treatment of Cancer QLQ-C30: a quality-of-life instrument for use in international clinical trials in oncology. *J Natl Cancer Inst.*, 1993, 3, 85(5), 365-76.

[2] Acharya, S; Bhat, PV; Acharya, S. Factors affecting oral health-related quality of life among pregnant women. *Int. J. Dent Hyg.*, 2009, 7(2), 102-7.

[3] Acharya, S. Oral health-related quality of life and its associated factors in an Indian adult population. *Oral Health Prev Dent.*, 2008, 6(3), 175-84.

[4] Adulyanon, S; Sheiham, A. Oral impact on daily performances: measuring oral health and quality of life. In: Slade GD, editor. Measuring oral health and quality of life. Chapel Hill, NC: Dept. of Dental Ecology, School of Dentistry, University of North Carolina, 1997. 151-60.

[5] Agou, S; Malhotra, M; Tompson, B; Prakash, P; Locker, D. Is the child oral health quality of life questionnaire sensitive to change in the context of orthodontic treatment? A brief communication. *J Public Health Dent*, 2008, 68(4), 246-8.

[6] Al Habashneh, R; Khader, YS; Salameh, S. Use of the Arabic version of Oral Health Impact Profile-14 to evaluate the impact of periodontal disease on oral health-related quality of life among Jordanian adults. *J Oral Sci.*, 2012, 54(1), 113-20.

[7] Albashaireh, ZS; Alhusein, AA; ashdeh, MM. Clinical assessments and patient evaluations of the esthetic quality of maxillary anterior restorations. *Int. J. Prosthodont.*, 2009, 22(1), 65-71.

[8] Albornoz, CR; Pusic, AL; Reavey, P; Scott, AM; Klassen, AF; Cano, SJ; Cordeiro, PG; Matros, E. Measuring health-related quality of life outcomes in head and neck reconstruction. *Clin Plast Surg.*, 2013, 40(2), 341-9.

[9] Al-Harthi, LS; Cullinan, MP; Leichter, JW; Thomson, WM. The impact of periodontitis on oral health-related quality of life: a review of the evidence from observational studies. *Aust Dent J.*, 2013, 58(3), 274-7.

[10] Allen, F; Locker, D. A modified short version of the oral health impact profile for assessing health-related quality of life in edentulous adults. *Int. J. Prosthodont*, 2002, 15(5), 446-50.

[11] Allen, PF; O'Sullivan, M; Locker, D. Determining the minimally important difference for the Oral Health Impact Profile-20. *Eur J Oral Sci*, 2009, 117(2), 129-34.

[12] Allen, PF. Assessment of oral health related quality of life. *Health Qual Life Outcomes.*, 2003, 1, 40.

[13] Allison, PJ; Locker, D; Feine, JS. Quality of life: a dynamic construct. *Soc Sci Med.*, 1997, 45(2), 221-30.

[14] Amato, JN; Barbosa, TS; Kobayashi, FY; Gavião, MB. Changes in the oral-health-related quality of life of Brazilian children after an educational preventive programme: an 1-month longitudinal evaluation. *Int. J. Dent Hyg*., 2014, 12(3), 226-33.

[15] Andresen, EM; Catlin, TK; Wyrwich, KW; Jackson-Thompson, J. Retest reliability of surveillance questions on health related quality of life. *J Epidemiol Community Health*, 2003, 57(5), 339-43.

[16] Araújo, AC; Gusmão, ES; Batista, JE; Cimões, R. Impact of periodontal disease on quality of life. *Quintessence Int.*, 2010, 41(6), e111-8.

[17] Aslund, M; Suvan, J; Moles, DR; D'Aiuto, F; Tonetti, MS. Effects of two different methods of non-surgical periodontal therapy on patient perception of pain and quality of life: a randomized controlled clinical trial. *J Periodontol.*, 2008, 79(6), 1031-40.

[18] Åstrøm, AN; Ekback, G; Ordell, S; Nasir, E. Long-term routine dental attendance: influence on tooth loss and oral health-related quality of life in Swedish older adults. *Community Dent Oral Epidemiol.*, 2014, 42(5), 460-9.

[19] Åstrøm, AN; Okullo, I. Validity and reliability of the Oral Impacts on Daily Performance (OIDP) frequency scale: a cross-sectional study of adolescents in Uganda. *BMC Oral Health*, 2003, 3(1), 5.

[20] Atchison, KA; Dolan, TA. Development of the Geriatric Oral Health Assessment Index. *J Dent Educ*, 1990, 54(11), 680-7.

[21] Baiardini, I; Bousquet, PJ; Brzoza, Z; Canonica, GW; Compalati, E; Fiocchi, A; Fokkens, W; van Wijk, RG; La, Grutta, S; Lombardi, C; Maurer, M; Pinto, AM; Ridolo, E; Senna, GE; Terreehorst, I; Todo Bom, A; Bousquet, J; Zuberbier, T; Braido, F. Recommendations for assessing Patient-Reported Outcomes and Health-Related quality of life in clinical trials on allergy: a GA2LEN taskforce position paper. *Allergy*, 2010, 65, 290–295.

[22] Bakas, T; McLennon, SM; Carpenter, JS; Buelow, JM; Otte, JL; Hanna, KM; Ellett, ML; Hadler, KA; Welch, JL. Systematic review of health-related quality of life models. *Health Qual Life Outcomes.*, 2012, 10, 134.

[23] Baker, SR; Pankhurst, CL; Robinson, PG. Utility of two oral health-related quality-of-life measures in patients with xerostomia. *Community Dent Oral Epidemiol*, 2006, 34(5), 351-62.

[24] Baker, SR. Testing a conceptual model of oral health: a structural equation modeling approach. *J Dent Res*, 2007, 86(8), 708-12.

[25] Barbosa, TS; Tureli, MC; Gavião, MB. Validity and reliability of the Child Perceptions Questionnaires applied in Brazilian children. *BMC Oral Health.*, 2009, 9, 13.

[26] Barer, GM; Gurevich, KG; Smirniagina, VV; Fabrikant, EG. [Validation of Oral Health Impact Profile (OHIP) quality of life questionnaire in Russian patients with evidence of chronic generalized periodontitis]. *Stomatologiia (Mosk).*, 2007, 86(5), 27-30.

[27] Batista, M; Lawrence, H; Rosário, de, Sousa, M. Impact of tooth loss related to number and position on oral health quality of life among adults. *Health Qual Life Outcomes.*, 2014, 12(1), 165.

[28] Batista, MJ; Perianes, LB; Hilgert, JB; Hugo, FN; Sousa, Mda, L. The impacts of oral health on quality of life in working adults. *Braz Oral Res.*, 2014, 28(1).

[29] Bergner, M; Bobbitt, RA; Carter, WB; Gilson, BS. The Sickness Impact Profile: development and final revision of a health status measure. *Med Care*, 1981, 19(8), 787-805.

[30] Bernabe, E; de Oliveira, CM; Sheiham, A; Tsakos, G. Comparison of the generic and condition-specific forms of the oral impacts on daily performances (OIDP) index. *J Public Health Dent*, 2009, 69, 176-81.

[31] Bernabé, E; de Oliveira, CM; Sheiham, A. Comparison of the discriminative ability of a generic and a condition-specific OHRQoL measure in adolescents with and without normative need for orthodontic treatment. *Health Qual Life Outcomes*, 2008, 21, 64.

[32] Bernabe, E; Sheiham, A; Tsakos, G. A comprehensive evaluation of the validity of Child-OIDP: further evidence from Peru. *Community Dent Oral Epidemiol*, 2008, 36(4), 317-25.

[33] Bernabé, E,cenes, W. Periodontal disease and quality of life in British adults. *J. Clin. Periodontol.*, 2010, 37(11), 968-72.

[34] Blanc, J; Boyer, L; Le Coz, P; Auquier, P. Metacognition: towards a new approach to quality of life. *Qual Life Res.*, 2014, 23(2), 467–75.

[35] Boodhwani, M; Andelfinger, G; Leipsic, J; Lindsay, T; McMurtry, MS; Therrien, J; Siu, SC;, Canadian, Cardiovascular, Society. Canadian Cardiovascular Society position statement on the management of thoracic aortic disease. *Can. J. Cardiol.*, 2014, 30(6), 577-89.

[36] Bourgeois, DM; Lodra, JC. European global oral health indicators development project. Report Proceedings. Paris, FR: Quintessence International, 2004.

[37] Bower, JE; Bak, K; Berger, A; Breitbart, W; Escalante, CP; Ganz, PA; Schnipper, HH; Lacchetti, C; Ligibel, JA; Lyman, GH; Ogaily, MS; Pirl, WF; Jacobsen, PB;, American, Society, of, Clinical, Oncology. Screening, assessment, and management of fatigue in adult survivors of cancer: an American Society of Clinical oncology clinical practice guideline adaptation. *J. Clin. Oncol.*, 2014, 10, 32(17), 1840-50.

[38] Brauchle, F; Noack, M; Reich, E. Impact of periodontal disease and periodontal therapy on oral health-related quality of life. *Int Dent J.*, 2013, 63(6), 306-11.

[39] Brennan, DS; Spencer, AJ; Roberts-Thomson, KF. Quality of life and disability weights associated with periodontal disease. *J Dent Res.*, 2007, 86(8), 713-7.

[40] Broder, HL; Wilson-Genderson, M; Sischo, L. Reliability and validity testing for the Child Oral Health Impact Profile-Reduced (COHIP-SF 19). *J Public Health Dent.*, 2012, 72(4), 302-12.

[41] Broder, HL. Children's oral health-related quality of life. *Community Dent Oral Epidemiol*, 2007, 35 Suppl 1, 5-7.

[42] Brondani, MA; MacEntee, MI. The concept of validity in sociodental indicators and oral health-related quality-of-life measures. *Community Dent Oral Epidemiol.*, 2007, 35(6), 472-8.

[43] Brondani, MA; MacEntee, MI. Thirty years of portraying oral health through models: what have we accomplished in oral health-related quality of life research? *Qual Life Res.*, 2014, 23(4), 1087-96.

[44] Burke, FJ; Busby, M; McHugh, S; Delargy, S; Mullins, A; Matthews, R. Evaluation of an oral health scoring system by dentists in general dental practice. *Br Dent J*, 2003, 194(4), 215-8, discussion 05.

[45] Bush, L; Horenkamp, N; Morley, J; Spiro, A. D-E-N-T-A-L: a rapid self-administered screening instrument to promote referrals for further evaluation in older adults. *J Am Geriatr Soc*, 1996, 44(8), 979-81.

[46] Cagney, KA; Wu, AW; Fink, NE; Jenckes, MW; Meyer, KB; Bass, EB; Powe, NR. Formal literature review of quality-of-life instruments used in end-stage renal disease. *Am. J. Kidney Dis*, 2000, 36, 327–336.

[47] Castro, RA; Cortes, MI; Leao, AT; Portela, MC; Souza, IP; Tsakos, G; et al., Child-OIDP index in Brazil: cross-cultural adaptation and validation. *Health Qual Life Outcomes*, 2008, 6, 68.

[48] Cella, D; Nowinski, CJ. Measuring quality of life in chronic illness: the functional assessment of chronic illness therapy measurement system. *Arch Phys Med Rehabil.*, 2002, 83(12 Suppl 2), S10-7.

[49] Cella, D; Yount, S; Rothrock, N; Gershon, R; Cook, K; Reeve, B; et al., On behalf of the PROMIS cooperative group. The Patient Reported Outcomes Measurement Information System (PROMIS): Progress of an NIH Roadmap Cooperative Group during its first two years. *Medical Care*, 2007, 45(5), S3–S11.

[50] Cella, DF; Tulsky, DS; Gray, G; Sarafian, B; Linn, E; Bonomi, A; Silberman, M; Yellen, SB; Winicour, P; Brannon, J; et al., The Functional Assessment of Cancer Therapy scale: development and validation of the general measure. *J. Clin. Oncol.*, 1993, 11(3), 570-9.

[51] Cella, DF. Manual of the Functional Assessment of Chronic Illness Therapy measurement system (version 4). Northwestern: CORE Evanston Northwestern Healthcare and Northwestern University: 1997.

[52] Cornejo, C; Rossi, G; Rama, A; Gomez-Gutierrez, N; Alvaredo, G; Squassi, A; Klemonskis, G. Oral health status and oral health-related quality of life in pregnant women from socially deprived populations. *Acta Odontol Latinoam.*, 2013, 26(2), 68-74.

[53] Cornell, JE; Saunders, MJ; Paunovich, ED; Frisch, MD. Oral health quality of life inventory (OH-QoL). In: Slade GD, editor. Measuring oral health and quality of life. Chapel Hill, NC Dept. of Dental Ecology, School of Dentistry, University of North Carolina; 1997. 135-50.

[54] Costa, DS; King, MT. Conceptual, classification or causal: models of health status and health-related quality of life. *Expert Rev Pharmacoecon Outcomes Res.*, 2013, 13(5), 631-40.

[55] Cunha-Cruz, J; Hujoel, PP; Kressin, NR. Oral health-related quality of life of periodontal patients. *J Periodontal Res.*, 2007, 42(2), 169-76.

[56] Cunningham, SJ; Garratt, AM; Hunt, NP. Development of a condition-specific quality of life measure for patients with dentofacial deformity: I. Reliability of the instrument. *Community Dent Oral Epidemiol*, 2000, 28(3), 195-201.

[57] Cushing, AM; Sheiham, A; Maizels, J. Developing socio-dental indicators--the social impact of dental disease. *Community Dent Health*, 1986, 3(1), 3-17.

[58] Dable, RA; Nazirkar, GS; Singh, SB; Wasnik, PB. Assessment of Oral Health Related Quality of Life Among Completely Edentulous Patients in Western India by Using GOHAI. *J. Clin. Diagn Res.*, 2013, 7(9), 2063-7.

[59] Dable, RA; Yashwante, BJ; athe, SS; Gaikwad, BS; Patil, PB; Momin, AA. Tooth loss--how emotional it is for the elderly in India? *Oral Health Dent Manag.*, 2014, 13(2), 305-10.

[60] De, Maeyer, J; Vanderplasschen, W; Broekaert, E. Quality of life among opiate-dependent individuals: A review of the literature. *Int. J. Drug Policy*, 2010.

[61] DeBaz, C; Shamia, H; Hahn, J; Mithani, S; Sadeghi, G; Palomo, L. Periodontitis impacts quality of life in postmenopausal women. *Climacteric.*, 2015, 10, 1-6.

[62] Dechi, RJ; Leal, AF; Padilha, DM; Brondani, MA. Vulnerability and the psychosocial aspects of tooth loss in old age: a Southern Brazilian study. *J Cross Cult Gerontol.*, 2012, 27(3), 239-58.

[63] Del, Fabbro, M; Taschieri, S; Weinstein, R. Quality of life after microscopic periradicular surgery using two different incision techniques: a randomized clinical study. *Int Endod J.*, 2009, 42(4), 360-7.

[64] Dolan, TA; Gooch, BF; Bourque, LB. Associations of self-reported dental health and general health measures in the Rand Health Insurance Experiment. *Community Dent Oral Epidemiol*, 1991, 19(1), 1-8.

[65] Dolan, TA; Peek, CW; Stuck, AE; Beck, JC. Three-year changes in global oral health rating by elderly dentate adults. *Community Dent Oral Epidemiol*, 1998, 26(1), 62-9.

[66] Dumitrescu, AL; Dogaru, BC; Dogaru, CD. Self-control and self-confidence: their relationship to self-rated oral health status and behaviours. *Oral Health Prev Dent.*, 2009b, 7(2), 155-62.

[67] Dumitrescu, AL; Dogaru, CB; Duţă, C; Manolescu, B. Body weight, shame, guilt and oral health: a path analysis model in undergraduate students. *Rom J Intern Med.*, 2011b, 49(4), 281-8.

[68] Dumitrescu, AL; Kawamura, M; Dogaru, B; Dogaru, C. Investigating the relationship between self-reported oral health status, oral health-related behaviours and self-consciousness in Romania. *Oral Health Prev Dent.*, 2008a, 6(2), 95-103.

[69] Dumitrescu, AL; Kawamura, M; Toma, C; Lascu, V. Social desirability, social intelligence and self-rated oral health status and behaviours. *Rom J Intern Med.*, 2007a, 45(4), 393-400.

[70] Dumitrescu, AL; Kawamura, M. Involvement of psychosocial factors in the association of obesity with periodontitis. *J Oral Sci.*, 2010, 52(1), 115-24.

[71] Dumitrescu, AL; Toma, C; Lascu, V; Lascu, B. The interplay of attention and self-monitoring with self-reporting oral health. *Rom J Intern Med.*, 2011a, 49(2), 129-36.

[72] Dumitrescu, AL; Toma, C; Lascu, V. Investigating the use of specific cognitive emotion regulation strategies in response to the experience of gingival bleeding. *Rom J Intern Med.*, 2011c, 49(3), 207-15.

[73] Dumitrescu, AL; Toma, C; Lascu, V. Self-liking, self-competence, body investment and perfectionism: associations with oral health status and oral-health-related behaviours. *Oral Health Prev Dent.*, 2009a, 7(2), 191-200.

[74] Dumitrescu, AL; Zetu, L; Teslaru, S; Dogaru, BC; Dogaru, CD. Is it an association between body appreciation, self-criticism, oral health status and oral health-related behaviors? *Rom J Intern Med.*, 2008b, 46(4), 343-50.

[75] Dumitrescu, AL. Investigating the relationship between self-reported oral health status, oral health-related behaviors, type A behavior pattern, perceived stress and emotional intelligence. *Rom J Intern Med.*, 2007b, 45(1), 67-76.

[76] Durham, J; Fraser, HM; McCracken, GI; Stone, KM; John, MT; Preshaw, PM. Impact of periodontitis on oral health-related quality of life. *J Dent.*, 2013, 41(4), 370-6.

[77] Eltas, A; Uslu, MÖ. Evaluation of oral health-related quality-of-life in patients with generalized aggressive periodontitis. *Acta Odontol Scand.*, 2013-Jul, 71(3-4), 547-52.
[78] Emami, E; Thomason, JM. In individuals with complete tooth loss, the mandibular implant-retained overdenture increases patient satisfaction and oral health related quality of life compared to conventional dentures. *J Evid Based Dent Pract.*, 2013, 13(3), 94-6.
[79] Feitosa, S; Colares, V; Pinkham, J. The psychosocial effects of severe caries in 4-year-old children in Recife, Pernambuco, Brazil. *Cad Saúde Pública*, 2005, 21, 1550-6.
[80] Ferrans, CE; Powers, M. Psychometric assessment of the Quality of Life Index. *Res Nurs Health*, 1992, 15, 29–38.
[81] Ferrans, CE; Zerwic, JJ; Wilbur, JE; Larson, JL. Conceptual model of health-related quality of life. *J Nurs Scholarsh*, 2005, 37(4), 336–342.
[82] Ferrans, CE. Definitions and conceptual models of quality of life. In: Lipscomb J, Gotay CC, Snyder C, editors. Outcomes assessment in cancer. Cambridge, England: Cambridge University; 2005. 14–30.
[83] Franke, M; Bröseler, F; Tietmann, C. Patient-related Evaluation After Systematic Periodontal Therapy - A Clinical Study on Periodontal Health-related Quality of Life (PHQoL). *Oral Health Prev Dent.*, 2014 10.
[84] Gadbdury-Amyot, CC; Williams, KB; Krust-Bray, K; Manne, D; Collins, P. Validity and reliability of the oral health-related quality of life instrument for dental hygiene. *J Dent Hygiene*, 1999, 73, 126–34.
[85] Gerritsen, AE; Allen, PF; Witter, DJ; Bronkhorst, EM; Creugers, NH. Tooth loss and oral health-related quality of life: a systematic review and meta-analysis. *Health Qual Life Outcomes.*, 2010, 5, 8, 126.
[86] Gherunpong, S; Tsakos, G; Sheiham, A. Developing and evaluating an oral health related quality of life index for children: The Child-OIDP. *Community Dent Health*, 2004, 21, 161–9.
[87] Gilbert, GH; Duncan, RP; Heft, MW; Dolan, TA; Vogel, WB. Multidimensionality of Oral Health in Dentate Adults. *Medical Care*, 1998, 36(7), 988-1001.
[88] Gilbert, GH; Heft, MW; Duncan, RP. Oral signs, symptoms, and behaviors in older Floridians. *J Public Health Dent*, 1993, 53(3), 151-7.
[89] Gilchrist, F; Rodd, H; Deery, C,shman, Z. Assessment of the quality of measures of child oral health-related quality of life. *BMC Oral Health.*, 2014, 23, 14, 40.
[90] Gil-Montoya, JA; de Mello, AL; Barrios, R; Gonzalez-Moles, MA; Bravo, M. Oral health in the elderly patient and its impact on general well-being: a nonsystematic review. *Clin Interv Aging.*, 2015, 11, 10, 461-7.
[91] Gomes, AS; Abegg, C. [The impact of oral health on daily performance of municipal waste disposal workers in Porto Alegre, Rio Grande do Sul State,Brazil]. *Cad Saude Publica.*, 2007, 23(7), 1707-14.
[92] Gülcan, F; Nasir, E; Ekbäck, G; Ordell, S; Åstrøm, AN. Change in Oral Impacts on Daily Performances (OIDP) with increasing age: testing the evaluative properties of the OIDP frequency inventory using prospective data from Norway and Sweden. *BMC Oral Health.*, 2014, 31, 14, 59.
[93] Guyatt, GH; Feeny, DH; Patrick, DL. Measuring health-related quality of life. *Ann Intern Med*, 1993, 118(8), 622-9.

[94] Halyard, MY; Ferrans, CE. Quality-of-Life assessment for routine oncology clinical practice. *J Support Oncol.*, 2008, 6(5), 221-9, 233.

[95] Haywood, K; Garratt, A; Fitzpatrick, R. Quality of life in older people: a structured review of generic self-assessed health instruments. *Quality Life Res*, 14, 1651–1668, 2005

[96] Haywood, KL; Garratt, AM; Fitzpatrick, R. Older people specific health status and quality of life: a structured review of self-assessed instruments. *J Eval Clin Pract.*, 2005, 11(4), 315-27.

[97] Haywood, KL; Garratt, AM; Fitzpatrick, R. Quality of life in older people: a structured review of self-assessed health instruments. *Expert Rev Pharmacoecon Outcomes Res.*, 2006, 6(2), 181-94.

[98] Haywood, KL; Garratt, AM; Fitzpatrick, R. Quality of life in older people: a structured review of generic self-assessed health instruments. *Qual Life Res.*, 2005, 14(7), 1651-68.

[99] Hebling, E; Pereira, AC. Oral health-related quality of life: a critical appraisal of assessment tools used in elderly people. *Gerodontology.*, 2007, 24(3), 151-61.

[100] Hennessy, CH; Moriarty, DG; Zack, MM; Scherr, PA; Brackbill, R. Measuring health-related quality of life for public health surveillance. *Public Health Rep*, 1994, 109(5), 665-72.

[101] Huang, DL; Park, M. Socioeconomic and racial/ethnic oral health disparities among US older adults: oral health quality of life and dentition. *J Public Health Dent.*, 2014 18.

[102] Hultin, M; Davidson, T; Gynther, G; Helgesson, G; Jemt, T; Lekholm, U; Nilner, K; Nordenram, G; Norlund, A; Rohlin, M; Sunnegardh-Gronberg, K; Tranaeus, S. Oral rehabilitation of tooth loss: a systematic review of quantitative studies of OHRQoL. *Int. J. Prosthodont.*, 2012, 25(6), 543-52.

[103] Humphris, G; Freeman, R; Gibson, B; Simpson, K; Whelton, H. Oral health-related quality of life for 8-10-year-old children: an assessment of a new measure. *Community Dent Oral Epidemiol.*, 2005, 33(5), 326-32.

[104] Inglehart, M. Oral health and quality of life. In: Mostofsky D, Forgione A, Giddon D, editors. Behavioral Dentistry. Oxford: Blackwell Munkgard, 2006. 19-28.

[105] International Society for Quality of Life Research (prepared by Aaronson N, Choucair A, Elliott T, Greenhalgh J, Halyard M, Hess R, Miller D, Reeve B, Santana M, Snyder C. User's Guide to Implementing Patient-Reported Outcomes Assessment in Clinical Practice, Version: December 11, 2011.

[106] Irfan, UM; Dawson, DV; Bissada, NF. Epidemiology of periodontal disease: a review and clinical perspectives. *J Int Acad Periodontol.*, 2001, 3, 14–21.

[107] Irvine, EJ. Quality of Life - rationale and methods for developing a disease-specific instrument for inflammatory bowel disease. *Scand J Gastroenterol Suppl*, 1993, 199, 22-7.

[108] Jansson, H; Wahlin, Å; Johansson, V; Åkerman, S; Lundegren, N; Isberg, PE; Norderyd, O. Impact of periodontal disease experience on oral health-related quality of life. *J Periodontol.*, 2014, 85(3), 438-45.

[109] Johannsen, A; Westergren, A; Johannsen, G. Dental implants from the patients perspective: transition from tooth loss, through amputation to implants - negative and positive trajectories. *J. Clin. Periodontol.*, 2012, 39(7), 681-7.

[110] John, MT; LeResche, L; Koepsell, TD; Hujoel, P; Miglioretti, DL; Micheelis, W. Oral health-related quality of life in Germany. *Eur J Oral Sci.*, 2003, 111(6), 483-91.

[111] John, MT. Exploring dimensions of oral health-related quality of life using experts' opinions. *Qual Life Res*, 2007, 16(4), 697-704.

[112] Jokovic, A; Locker, D; Guyatt, G. How well do parents know their children? Implications for proxy reporting of child health-related quality of life. *Qual Life Res*, 2004, 13(7), 1297-307.

[113] Jokovic, A; Locker, D; Stephens, M; Kenny, D; Tompson, B; Guyatt, G. Measuring parental perceptions of child oral health-related quality of life. *J Public Health Dent.*, 2003 Spring, 63(2), 67-72.

[114] Jokovic, A; Locker, D; Stephens, M; Kenny, D; Tompson, B; Guyatt, G. Validity and reliability of a questionnaire for measuring child oral-health-related quality of life *J Dent Res*, 2002a, 81(7), 459-63.

[115] Jokovic, A; Locker, D; Tompson, B; Guyatt, G. Questionnaire for measuring oral health related quality of life in eight- to ten-year-old children. *Pediatr Dent*, 2004, 26(6), 512-8.

[116] Jones, JA; Kressin, NR; Miller, DR; Orner, MB; Garcia, RI; Spiro, A, 3rd. Comparison of patient-based oral health outcome measures. *Qual Life Res.*, 2004, 13(5), 975-85.

[117] Jones, JA; Orner, MB; Spiro, A 3rd; Kressin, NR. Tooth loss and dentures: patients' perspectives. *Int Dent J*, 2003, 53(5 Suppl), 327-34.

[118] Jönsson, B; Öhrn, K. Evaluation of the effect of non-surgical periodontal treatment on oral health-related quality of life: estimation of minimal important differences 1 year after treatment. *J. Clin. Periodontol.*, 2014, 41(3), 275-82.

[119] Jowett, AK; Orr, MT; Rawlinson, A; Robinson, PG. Psychosocial impact of periodontal disease and its treatment with 24-h root surface debridement. *J. Clin. Periodontol.*, 2009, 36(5), 413-8.

[120] Karlsson, E; Lymer, UB; Hakeberg, M. Periodontitis from the patient's perspective, a qualitative study. *Int. J. Dent Hyg.*, 2009, 7(1), 23-30.

[121] Kimura, A; Arakawa, H; Noda, K; Yamazaki, S; Hara, ES; Mino, T; Matsuka, Y; Mulligan, R; Kuboki, T. Response shift in oral health-related quality of life measurement in patients with partial edentulism. *J Oral Rehabil.*, 2012, 39(1), 44-54.

[122] Kressin, N; Spiro, A 3rd; Bosse, R; Garcia, R; Kazis, L. Assessing oral health-related quality of life: findings from the normative aging study. *Med Care*, 1996, 34(5), 416-27.

[123] Krisdapong, S; Prasertsom, P; Rattanarangsima, K; Adulyanon, S; Sheiham, A. Setting oral health goals that include oral health-related quality of life measures: a study carried out among adolescents in Thailand. *Cad Saude Publica.*, 2012, 28(10), 1881-92.

[124] Krisdapong, S; Prasertsom, P; Rattanarangsima, K; Adulyanon, S; Sheiham, A. Using associations between oral diseases and oral health-related quality of life in a nationally representative sample to propose oral health goals for 12-year-old children in Thailand. *Int Dent J.*, 2012b, 62(6), 320-30.

[125] Krisdapong, S; Prasertsom, P; Rattanarangsima, K; Adulyanon, S; Sheiham, A. Setting oral health goals that include oral health-related quality of life measures: a study carried out among adolescents in Thailand. *Cad Saude Publica.*, 2012c, 28(10), 1881-92.

[126] Krisdapong, S; Prasertsom, P; Rattanarangsima, K; Sheiham, A; Tsakos, G. The impacts of gingivitis and calculus on Thai children's quality of life. *J. Clin. Periodontol.*, 2012d, 39(9), 834-43.

[127] Krisdapong, S; Prasertsom, P; Rattanarangsima, K; Sheiham, A. Relationships between oral diseases and impacts on Thai schoolchildren's quality of life: evidence from a Thai national oral health survey of 12- and 15-year-olds. *Community Dent Oral Epidemiol.*, 2012a, 40(6), 550-9.

[128] Lawrence, HP; Thomson, WM; Broadbent, JM; Poulton, R. Oral health-related quality of life in a birth cohort of 32-year olds. *Community Dent Oral Epidemiol.*, 2008, 36(4), 305-16.

[129] Leao, A; Sheiham, A. The development of a socio-dental measure of dental impacts on daily living. *Community Dent Health*, 1996, 13(1), 22-6.

[130] Li, S; Veronneau, J; Allison, PJ. Validation of a French language version of the Early Childhood Oral Health Impact Scale (ECOHIS). *Health Qual Life Outcomes*, 2008, 6, 9.

[131] Li, Z; Zhu, L; Sha, Y. [Effects of periodontal health and related factors on the oral health-related quality of life in type 2 diabetic patients with chronic periodontitis]. *Hua Xi Kou Qiang Yi Xue Za Zhi.*, 2011, 29(4), 379-83.

[132] Locker, D; Allen, F. What do measures of 'oral health-related quality of life' measure?. *Community Dent Oral Epidemiol*, 2007, 35, 401–411.

[133] Locker, D; Allen, PF. Developing short-form measures of oral health-related quality of life. *J Public Health Dent*, 2002, 62(1), 13-20.

[134] Locker, D; Berka, E; Jokovic, A; Tompson, B. Does self-weighting of items enhance the performance of an oral health-related quality of life questionnaire? *Community Dent Oral Epidemiol*, 2007, 35(1), 35-43.

[135] Locker, D; Jokovic, A; Clarke, M. Assessing the responsiveness of measures of oral health related quality of life *Community Dent Oral Epidemiol*, 2004, 32(1), 10-8.

[136] Locker, D; Jokovic, A; Stephens, M; Kenny, D; Tompson, B; Guyatt, G. Family impact of child oral and oro-facial conditions. *Community Dent Oral Epidemiol.*, 2002, 30(6), 438-48.

[137] Locker, D; Miller, Y. Evaluation of subjective oral health status indicators. *J Public Health Dent*, 1994, 54, 167–76.

[138] Locker, D; Miller, Y. Subjectively reported oral health status in an adult population. *Community Dent Oral Epidemiol*, 1994, 22(6), 425-30.

[139] Locker, D. Validity of single-item parental ratings of child oral health. *Int. J. Paediatr Dent*, 2008, 18(6), 407-14.

[140] López, R; Baelum, V. Oral health impact of periodontal diseases in adolescents. *J Dent Res.*, 2007, 86(11), 1105-9.

[141] MacEntee, MI. An existential model of oral health from evolving views on health, function and disability. *Community Dent Health.*, 2006, 23(1), 5-14.

[142] Mariño, R; Schofield, M; Wright, C; Calache, H; Minichiello, V. Self-reported and clinically determined oral health status predictors for quality of life in dentate older migrant adults. *Community Dent Oral Epidemiol.*, 2008, 36(1), 85-94.

[143] Marinus, J; Ramaker, C; van Hilten, JJ; Stiggelbout, AM. Health related quality of life in Parkinson's disease: a systematic review of disease specific instruments. *J Neurol Neurosurg Psychiatry*, 2002, 72(2), 241-8.

[144] Marshman, Z; Rodd, H; Stern, M; Mitchell, C; Locker, D; Jokovic, A; Robinson, PG. An evaluation of the Child Perceptions Questionnaire in the UK. *Community Dent Health.*, 2005, 22(3), 151-5.

[145] Masood, M; Masood, Y; Saub, R; Newton, JT. Need of minimal important difference for oral health-related quality of life measures. *J Public Health Dent.*, 2014, 74(1), 13-20.

[146] Mathur, VP; Dhillon, JK; Logani, A; Agarwal, R. Development and validation of oral health-related early childhood quality of life tool for North Indian preschool children. *Indian J Dent Res.*, 2014, 25(5), 559-66.

[147] McGrath, C; Bedi, R. An evaluation of a new measure of oral health related quality of life-OHQoL-UK(W). *Community Dent Health*, 2001, 18(3), 138-43.

[148] McGrath, C; Bedi, R. Measuring the impact of oral health on life quality in two national surveys - functionalist versus hermeneutic approaches. *Community Dent Oral Epidemiol.*, 2002, 30(4), 254-9.

[149] McKenna, G; Allen, PF; Woods, N; O'Mahony, D; DaMata, C; Cronin, M; Normand, C. A preliminary report of the cost-effectiveness of tooth replacement strategies for partially dentate elders. *Gerodontology.*, 2013, 30(3), 207-13.

[150] Montero, J; Bravo, M; Albaladejo, A. Validation of two complementary oral-health related quality of life indicators (OIDP and OSS 0-10) in two qualitativelydistinct samples of the Spanish population. *Health Qual Life Outcomes.*, 2008, 18, 6, 101.

[151] Musurlieva, N; Stoykova, M; Boyadjiev, D. Validation of a scale assessing the impact of periodontal diseases on patients' quality of life in Bulgaria (pilot research). *Braz Dent J.*, 2012, 23(5), 570-4.

[152] Nagarajan, S; Chandra, RV. Perception of oral health related quality of life (OHQoL-UK) among periodontal risk patients before and after periodontal therapy. *Community Dent Health.*, 2012, 29(1), 90-4.

[153] Nanayakkara, V; Renzaho, A; Oldenburg, B; Ekanayake, L. Ethnic and socio-economic disparities in oral health outcomes and quality of life among Sri Lankan preschoolers: a cross-sectional study. *Int. J. Equity Health.*, 2013, 12, 89.

[154] Needleman, I; McGrath, C; Floyd, P; Biddle, A. Impact of oral health on the life quality of periodontal patients. *J. Clin. Periodontol.*, 2004, 31(6), 454-7.

[155] Ng, SK; Leung, WK. Oral health-related quality of life and periodontal status. *Community Dent Oral Epidemiol.*, 2006, 34(2), 114-22.

[156] Nguyen, TC; Witter, DJ; Bronkhorst, EM; Gerritsen, AE; Creugers, NH. Chewing ability and dental functional status. *Int. J. Prosthodont.*, 2011, 24(5), 428-36.

[157] Niesten, D; van Mourik, K; van der Sanden, W. The impact of having natural teeth on the QoL of frail dentulous older people. A qualitative study. *BMC Public Health.*, 2012, 2, 12, 839.

[158] O'Dowd, LK; Durham, J; McCracken, GI; Preshaw, PM. Patients' experiences of the impact of periodontal disease. *J. Clin. Periodontol.*, 2010, 37(4), 334-9.

[159] Ostberg, AL; Halling, A; Lindblad, U. A gender perspective of self-perceived oral health in adolescents: associations with attitudes and behaviours. *Community Dent Health.*, 2001, 18(2), 110-6.

[160] Ozcelik, O; Haytac, MC; Seydaoglu, G. Immediate post-operative effects of different periodontal treatment modalities on oral health-related quality of life: a randomized clinical trial. *J. Clin. Periodontol.*, 2007, 34(9), 788-96.

[161] Özhayat, EB; Gotfredsen, K. Oral health-related quality-of-life in patients to be treated with fixed or removable partial dental prostheses. *Acta Odontol Scand.*, 2013, 71(1), 113-9.

[162] Özhayat, EB. Influence of self-esteem and negative affectivity on oral health-related quality of life in patients with partial tooth loss. *Community Dent Oral Epidemiol.*, 2013, 41(5), 466-72.

[163] Pace-Balzan, A; Cawood, JI; Howell, R; Lowe, D; Rogers, SN. The Liverpool Oral Rehabilitation Questionnaire: a pilot study. *J Oral Rehabil*, 2004, 31(6), 609-17.

[164] Pahel, BT; Rozier, RG; Slade, GD. Parental perceptions of children's oral health: the Early Childhood Oral Health Impact Scale (ECOHIS). *Health Qual Life Outcomes*, 2007, 5, 6.

[165] Papapanou, PN. Periodontal diseases: epidemiology. *Ann Periodontol.*, 1996, 1, 1–36.

[166] Patrick, DL; Deyo, RA. Generic and disease-specific measures in assessing health status and quality of life. *Med Care*, 1989, 27(3Suppl), S217-32.

[167] Pattussi, MP; Olinto, MT; Hardy, R; Sheiham, A. Clinical, social and psychosocial factors associated with self-rated oral health in Brazilian adolescents. *Community Dent Oral Epidemiol*, 2007, 35(5), 377-86.

[168] Peres, MA; Antunes, JL; Boing, AF; Peres, KG; Bastos, JL. Skin colour is associated with periodontal disease in Brazilian adults: a population-based oral health survey. *J. Clin. Periodontol*, 2007, 34(3), 196-201.

[169] Pinho, S; Ciriaco, C; Faber, J; Lenza, MA. Impact of dental asymmetries on the perception of smile esthetics. *Am. J. Orthod Dentofacial Orthop.*, 2007, 132(6), 748-53.

[170] Pistorius, J; Horn, JG; Pistorius, A; Kraft, J. Oral health-related quality of life in patients with removable dentures. *Schweiz Monatsschr Zahnmed.* 2013, 123(11), 964-71, 955.

[171] Preciado, A; Del, Río, J; Lynch, CD; Castillo-Oyagüe, R. A new, short, specific questionnaire (QoLIP-10) for evaluating the oral health-related quality of life of implant-retained overdenture and hybrid prosthesis wearers. *J Dent.*, 2013, 41(9), 753-63.

[172] Reisine, ST; Fertig, J; Weber, J; Leder, S. Impact of dental conditions on patients' quality of life. *Community Dent Oral Epidemiol*, 1989, 17(1), 7-10.

[173] Reissmann, DR; Remmler, A; John, MT; Schierz, O; Hirsch, C. Impact of response shift on the assessment of treatment effects using the Oral Health Impact Profile. *Eur J Oral Sci.*, 2012, 120(6), 520-5.

[174] Ring, L; Höfer, S; Heuston, F; Harris, D; O'Boyle, CA. Response shift masks the treatment impact on patient reported outcomes (PROs): the example of individual quality of life in edentulous patients. *Health Qual Life Outcomes.*, 2005, 7, 3, 55.

[175] Riordain, RN; McCreary, C. The use of quality of life measures in oral medicine: a review of the literature. *Oral Dis.*, 2010, 16(5), 419-30.

[176] Robinson, PG; Nalweyiso, N; Busingye, J; Whitworth, J. Subjective impacts of dental caries and fluorosis in rural Ugandan children. *Community Dent Health.*, 2005, 22(4), 231-6.

[177] Rousseau, N; Steele, J; Exley, C. 'Your whole life is lived through your teeth': biographical disruption and experiences of tooth loss and replacement. *Sociol Health Illn.*, 2014, 36(3), 462-76.

[178] Saintrain, MV; de Souza, EH. Impact of tooth loss on the quality of life. *Gerodontology.*, 2012, 29(2), e632-6.

[179] Saito, A; Hosaka, Y; Kikuchi, M; Akamatsu, M; Fukaya, C; Matsumoto, S; Ueshima, F; Hayakawa, H; Fujinami, K; Nakagawa, T. Effect of initial periodontal therapy on oral health-related quality of life in patients with periodontitis in Japan. *J Periodontol.*, 2010, 81(7), 1001-9.

[180] Saito, A; Ota, K; Hosaka, Y; Akamatsu, M; Hayakawa, H; Fukaya, C; Ida, A; Fujinami, K; Sugito, H; Nakagawa, T. Potential impact of surgical periodontal therapy on oral health-related quality of life in patients with periodontitis: a pilot study. *J. Clin. Periodontol.*, 2011, 38(12), 1115-21.

[181] Salomon, JA; Nordhagen, S; Oza, S; Murray, CJ. Are Americans feeling less healthy? The puzzle of trends in self-rated health. *Am. J. Epidemiol*, 2009, 170(3), 343-51.

[182] Schwartz, CE; Sprangers, MA. Methodological approaches for assessing response shift in longitudinal health-related quality of-life research. *Soc Sci Med.*, 1999b, 48(11), 1531–48.

[183] Shanbhag, S; Dahiya, M; Croucher, R. The impact of periodontal therapy on oral health-related quality of life in adults: a systematic review. *J. Clin. Periodontol.*, 2012, 39(8), 725-35.

[184] Singh, KA; Brennan, DS. Chewing disability in older adults attributable to tooth loss and other oral conditions. *Gerodontology.*, 2012, 29(2), 106-10.

[185] Sisson, KL. Theoretical explanations for social inequalities in oral health. *Commun Dent Oral Epidemiol*, 2007, 35(2), 81-88.

[186] Slade, G. Measuring oral health and quality of life. Chapel Hill: 21. University of North Carolina, Dental Ecology; 1997.

[187] Slade, GD; Spencer, AJ; Locker, D; Hunt, RJ; Strauss, RP; Beck, JD. Variations in the social impact of oral conditions among older adults in South Australia, Ontario, and North Carolina. *J Dent Res*, 1996, 75(7), 1439-50.

[188] Slade, GD; Spencer, AJ. Development and evaluation of the Oral Health Impact Profile. *Community Dent Health*, 1994, 11(1), 3-11.

[189] Slade, GD. The oral health impact profile. In: Slade GD, editor. Measuring oral health and quality of life. Chapel Hill, NC: Dept. of Dental Ecology, School of Dentistry, University of North Carolina; 1997. 93-105.

[190] Smith, KW; Avis, NE; Assmann, SF. Distinguishing between quality of life and health status in quality of life research: a meta-analysis. *Qual Life Res.*, 1999, 8(5), 447-59.

[191] Somsak, K; Kaewplung, O. The effects of the number of natural teeth and posterior occluding pairs on the oral health-related quality of life in elderly dental patients. *Gerodontology.*, 2014, 6.

[192] Sprangers, MA; Schwartz, CE. Integrating response shift into health-related quality of life research: a theoretical model. *Soc Sci Med.*, 1999a, 48(11), 1507–15.

[193] Strauss, RP; Hunt, RJ. Understanding the value of teeth to older adults: influences on the quality of life. *J Am Dent Assoc*, 1993, 124(1), 105-10.

[194] Sugisaki, M; Kino, K; Yoshida, N; Ishikawa, T; Amagasa, T; Haketa, T. Development of a new questionnaire to assess pain-related limitations of daily functions in Japanese patients with temporomandibular disorders. *Community Dent Oral Epidemiol.*, 2005, 33(5), 384-95.

[195] Sundaram, NS; Narendar, R; Dineshkumar, P; Ramesh, SB; Gokulanathan, S. Evaluation of oral health related quality of life in patient with mild periodontitis among young male population of Namakkal district. *J Pharm Bioallied Sci.*, 2013, 5(Suppl 1), S30-2.

[196] Taichman, LS; Griggs, JJ; Inglehart, MR. Periodontal health, perceived oral health, and dental care utilization of breast cancer survivors. *J Public Health Dent.*, 2015, 3.

[197] Thomson, WM; Mejia, GC; Broadbent, JM; Poulton, R. Construct validity of Locker's global oral health item. *J Dent Res.*, 2012, 91(11), 1038-42.

[198] Tomazoni, F; Zanatta, FB; Tuchtenhagen, S; da, Rosa, GN; Del, Fabro, JP; Ardenghi, TM. Association of gingivitis with child oral health-related quality of life. *J Periodontol.*, 2014, 85(11), 1557-65.

[199] Tsakos, G; Bernabé, E; D'Aiuto, F; Pikhart, H; Tonetti, M; Sheiham, A; Donos, N. Assessing the minimally important difference in the oral impact on daily performances index in patients treated for periodontitis. *J. Clin. Periodontol*, 2010, 37(10), 903-9.

[200] Tsakos, G; Blair, YI; Yusuf, H; Wright, W; Watt, RG; Macpherson, LM. Developing a new self-reported scale of oral health outcomes for 5-year-old children (SOHO-5). *Health Qual Life Outcomes.*, 2012, 10, 62.

[201] Van, der, Geld, P; Oosterveld, P; van Heck, G; Kuijpers-Jagtman, AM. Smile attractiveness. Self-perception and influence on personality. *Angle Orthod.*, 2007, 77(5), 759-65.

[202] van, Nieuwenhuizen, C; Schene, AH; Koeter, MW; Huxley, PJ. The Lancashire Quality of Life Profile: modification and psychometric evaluation. *Soc Psychiatry Psychiatr Epidemiol*, 2001, 36(1), 36-44.

[203] Vanier, A; Leplège, A; Hardouin, JB; Sébille, V; Falissard, B. Semantic primes theory be helpful in designing questionnaires such as to prevent response shift. *J. Clin. Epidemiol.*, 2015, 31.

[204] Visscher, CM; Lobbezoo, F; Schuller, AA. Dental status and oral health-related quality of life. A population-based study. *J Oral Rehabil.*, 2014, 41(6), 416-22.

[205] Williams, KB; Gadbury-Amyot, CC; Bray, KK; Manne, D; Collins, P. Oral health-related quality of life: a model for dental hygiene. *J Dent Hyg.*, 1998 Spring, 72(2), 19-26.

[206] Wilson, IB; Cleary, PD. Linking clinical variables with health-related quality of life: A Conceptual model of patient outcomes. *JAMA*, 1995, 273(1), 59–65.

[207] Wong, RM; Ng, SK; Corbet, EF; Keung, Leung, W. Non-surgical periodontal therapy improves oral health-related quality of life. *J. Clin. Periodontol.*, 2012, 39(1), 53-61.

[208] World Health Organization. The World Health Organization Quality of Life assessment (WHOQoL): position paper from the World Health Organization. *Soc Sci Med*, 2005, 41(10):1403-1409.

[209] World Health Organization: International Classification of Functioning, disability, and Health: Children and Youth Version: ICF-CY. Geneva: World Health Organization; 2007.

[210] World Health Organization: International Classification of Functioning, Disability, and Health: ICF. Geneva: World Health Organization; 2001.

[211] World Health Organization: International Classification of Impairments, Disabilities, and Handicaps: A manual of classification relating to the consequences of disease. Geneva: World Health Organization; 1980.

[212] World Health Organization: The Constitution of the World Health Organization. Geneva, World Health Organization, 1947.

[213] Wu, AW; Fink, NE; Cagney, KA; Bass, EB; Rubin, HR; Meyer, KB; Sadler, JH; Powe, NR, Developing a health-related quality-of-life measure for end-stage renal disease: The CHOICE Health Experience Questionnaire. *Am. J. Kidney Dis.*, 2001, 37(1), 11-21.

[214] Yu, SJ; Chen, P; Zhu, GX. Relationship between implantation of missing anterior teeth and oral health-related quality of life. *Qual Life Res.*, 2013, 22(7), 1613-20.

[215] Zaitsu, T; Ueno, M; Shinada, K; Ohara, S; Wright, FA; Kawaguchi, Y. Association of clinical oral health status with self-rated oral health and GOHAI in Japanese adults. *Community Dent Health.*, 2011, 28(4), 297-300.

[216] Zanatta, FB; Ardenghi, TM; Antoniazzi, RP; Pinto, TM; Rösing, CK. Association between gingival bleeding and gingival enlargement and oral health-related quality of life (OHRQoL) of subjects under fixed orthodontic treatment: a cross-sectional study. *BMC Oral Health.*, 2012, 12, 53.

[217] Zhang, Q; Witter, DJ; Gerritsen, AE; Bronkhorst, EM; Creugers, NH. Functional dental status and oral health-related quality of life in an over 40 years old Chinese population. *Clin Oral Investig.*, 2013, 17(6), 1471-80.

In: Oral Health
Editor: Julia Renee Barnes

ISBN: 978-1-63482-832-1

Chapter III

Exploring the Relationship between Nutrition and Periodontal Disease

A. L. Dumitrescu*
Private practice, Bucharest, Romania

Abstract

Periodontal diseases are one of the common oral diseases and it is associated with formation of periodontal pockets, gingival abscesses, gingival recessions, tooth mobility, and finally teeth loss. The link between nutritional factors and periodontal disease has not been clearly established even if a highly number of studies has investigated this possible association. As periodontitis is associated with low serum/plasma micronutrient levels, it has been postulated that daily intake for vitamin C (ascorbic acid), vitamin E, zinc, lycopene, vitamin B, complex vitamin D, calcium, unsaturated fats and antioxidants would have useful adjunct benefits on the prevention and therapeutic management of periodontal disease. Regarding various beverages, the consumption of milk, coffee or green tea was also investigated in relationship with periodontitis. It has been showed that higher coffee consumption is associated with a significant reduction in number of teeth with periodontal bone loss, while green tea extract has been revealed to suppress the onset of loss of attachment and alveolar bone resorption in a rat model of experimental periodontitis. This chapter reviews the current knowledge in this research field, suggesting an adequate dietary advice for patients with chronic periodontitis.

1. Introduction

Periodontal diseases are one of the common oral diseases and it is associated with formation of periodontal pockets, gingival abscesses, gingival recessions, tooth mobility, and finally teeth loss. The link between nutritional factors and periodontal disease has not been

* E-mail: alexandrina_l_dumitrescu@yahoo.co.uk

clearly established even if a highly number of studies has investigated this possible association. This chapter reviews the current knowledge in this research field, suggesting an adequate dietary advice for patients with chronic periodontitis.

2. Definition of Terms

What is nutrition? According to *The Giessen Declaration* (2005), the following working definition of the current conventional science of nutrition as a biological discipline was adopted: "Nutrition science is ... the study of food systems, foods and drinks, and their nutrients and other constituents; and of their interactions within and between all relevant biological, social and environmental systems." "The purpose of nutrition science is to contribute to a world in which present and future generations fulfil their human potential, live in the best of health, and develop, sustain and enjoy an increasingly diverse human, living and physical environment." Moreover, it was stated that "Nutrition science should be the basis for food and nutrition policies. These should be designed to identify, create, conserve and protect rational, sustainable and equitable communal, national and global food systems, in order to sustain the health, well-being and integrity of humankind and also that of the living and physical worlds" (Leitzmann & Cannon, 2005; Beauman et al., 2005; Cannon & Leitzmann, 2005).

Dietary patterns can be characterized, according to the Scientific Report of the 2015 Dietary Guidelines Advisory Committee, in three main ways: 1) The first is by the use of an a priori index based on a set of dietary recommendations, such as the Healthy Eating Index (HEI)-2005 and 2010, the Alternate HEI (AHEI) and updated AHEI-2010, the Recommended Food Score (RFS), the Dietary Approaches to Stop Hypertension (DASH) score, the Mediterranean Diet Score (MDS), and the Alternate Mediterranean Diet Score (aMed); 2) The second method of dietary pattern assessment is through data-driven approaches, such as cluster (e.g. "Using the self-reported food and beverage intake data are there groups of people with distinct (non-overlapping) dietary patterns?") and factor analysis (e.g. "Which components of the diet track together to explain variations in food or beverage intake across diet patterns?") as well as outcome-dependent approaches are, such as reduced rank regression (e.g. "What combination of foods explains the most variation in one or more intermediate health markers?"); 3) The third method uses qualitative self-reported behaviors in aim to investigate participants' eating and drinking patterns, such as vegetarianism or ovo-lacto vegetarianism) (Dietary Guidelines Advisory Committee, 2015).

Malnutrition is an imbalance between the nutrients the body needs and the nutrients it gets. Thus, both **overnutrition** (defined as consumption of too many calories or too much of any specific nutrient—protein, fat, vitamin, mineral, or other dietary supplement), and **undernutrition** (defined as a disturbance of form or function arising from the deficiency of one or more nutrients) are forms of malnutrition (Beers & Berkow, 2004; Schenker, 2003). **Lack of nutrients** can result in deficiency syndromes (e.g. pellagra) and related disorders while excess intake of macronutrients can lead to obesity and related disorders (Beers & Berkow, 2004).

Food-based dietary guidelines (FBDG) are simple messages on healthy eating, indicating of what an individual should be intake in terms of foods rather than nutrients, as well as and offering to the general public a basic support to use when setting up meals or daily menus (WHO, 2003).

FBDG can be extensive and unspecific such as "eat plenty of fruits and vegetables," or more specific such as "eat five portions of fruits and vegetables a day" (WHO, 2003).

Messages may also indicate the type of food, such as "eat low fat dairy products and drink low fat milk," or be meal specific such as "eat breakfast every day" (EUFIC, 2009).

Dietary quality and **nutritional status** (defined as the extent to which nutrients are available to meet metabolic needs) (Wirt & Collins, 2009) are important for disease prevention and health promotion. However, associated with risk factors (e.g. smoking, lack of physical activity) nutrition may have a negative effect on the prevalence of several chronic diseases, such as cardiovascular disease, diabetes, obesity, cancers or osteoporosis.

3. Type of Nutrients

Macronutrients, such as carbohydrates, proteins (including essential amino acids), fats (including essential fatty acids), macrominerals, and water, represents the largeness part of the diet and supply energy and many essential nutrients. **Micronutrients** are represented by vitamins and minerals required in minute amounts (trace minerals) (Beers & Berkow, 2004). Nutrient-dense foods (e.g. vegetables, fruits, whole grains, fish, eggs, nuts, lean, low-fat forms of fluid milk, meat, and poultry prepared without added solid fats or sugars) are naturally rich in vitamins and minerals, retain naturally-occurring components such as fiber and are low in solid fats and without added solid fats, sugars, starches, or sodium (Beers & Berkow, 2004).

4. Current Reviews and Meta-Analyses Related on the Role of Nutrition in Periodontal Disease

Several reviews and meta-analyses have analyzed the impact of nutrition on periodontal health (Enwonwu et al., 2004; Enwonwu et al., 2002; Ritchie et al., 2002; Chapple, 2009; Van der Velden et al., 2011; Neiva et al., 2003; Johnson & Curtis, 1994; Bsoul & Terezhalmy, 2004; Enwonwu & Ritchie, 2007; Enwonwu, 1995; Sculley & Langley-Evans, 2002; Boyd & Lampi, 2001; Dorsky, 2001; Enwonwu, 1994; Boyd & Madden, 2003; Karp, 1994; Hornick, 2002; Van der Velden et al., 2011; Kulkarni et al., 2014).

The most recent systematic review, performed by Kulkarni et al., (2014), based on PubMed and Cochrane database literature search, concluded that:

> *"the link between nutrients and periodontal disease has not been clearly established. The published research reveals only a possible relationship between vitamins and minerals and periodontal disease. Vitamin E, zinc, lycopene and vitamin B complex may have useful adjunct benefits. However, there is inadequate evidence to link the nutritional status of the host to periodontal inflammation. More randomized controlled trials are needed to explore this association."*

A bi-directional relationship can be established between nutrition and periodontal disease and there is an increasing emphasis on their interrelationships (Figure 1.).

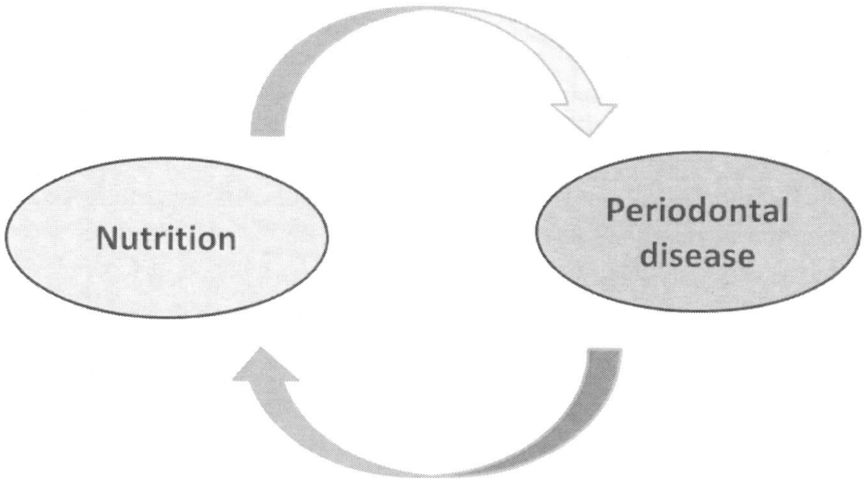

Figure 1. Inter-relationship between nutrition and periodontal disease.

5. Impact of Macronutrients on the Periodontal Disease Status

Macronutrients - are those nutrients required by the human body in large amounts (Tucker, 2010) (**Figure 2.**).

When *carbohydrates* roles are considered, we should consider that animal research has revealed the etiological role of dental plaque, as periodontal disease has been demonstrated to be induced in rats and in hamsters in relation to indigenous plaque (Crawford et al., 1978; Garant & Cho, 1979; Garant & Cho, 1980; Heijl et al., 1980; Wyss & Guggenheim, 1984; Lekic et al., 1989; Klausen, 1991; Yamazaki, 1992). A greater incidence of periodontitis lesions with active bone resorption was observed after 7 weeks in rats fed with a high-sucrose diet (Keyes' diet 2000) comparing with rats fed a normally laboratory chow diet (Garant & Cho, 1979; Garant & Cho, 1980). Moreover, when sucrose was added in the rats' diet (Heijl et al., 1980; Crawford et al., 1978; Abiko & Shimono, 1989) or in their drinking water (Lekic et al., 1989), it was revealed that a variety of microorganisms (e.g. *Streptococcus sobrinus*, *Actinomycesviscosus*, *Porphyromonas gingivalis*) can be established in rats that were fed with an ordinary food (Klausen, 1991). It was also reported that a diet with a smaller grain size is associated with less horizontal bone loss and periodontal bone support than a regular diet (Björnsson et al., 2003). The diet (e.g. sucrose-rich diet) seems also to be more the most consistent factor involved in the calculus formation in different strains of rats (Tanzer & Grant, 1993; Baer et al., 1967; Weinberg & Bral, 1999).

Few human studies have researched the potential role of dietary sugar in the etiology of periodontal disease. In an 3-week experimental period experimental gingivitis model in young adults, significantly higher levels of bleeding on probing scores were found when participants were fed with a diet high in carbohydrates when compared to those on a low sugar diet, even if no significant differences were observed with crevicular fluid flow and plaque amount (Sidi and Ashley, 1984). These findings have been further supported by a study performed by Baumgartner et al., (2009) who assessed the oral microbiota and clinical data in subjects without access to traditional oral hygiene methods and who ate a diet available in the Stone Age. The participants refrained from any oral hygiene measures and received a diet rich in fibre, anti-oxidants, and fish oils, but low in refined sugars and. Surprisingly, at week 4, even if dental plaque levels increased significantly (from 0.68 to 1.47, $P<0.001$) as well as the total bacterial count ($P<0.001$), mean bleeding on probing scores decreased (34.8% to 12.6%, $P<0.001$) (Baumgartner et al., 2009).

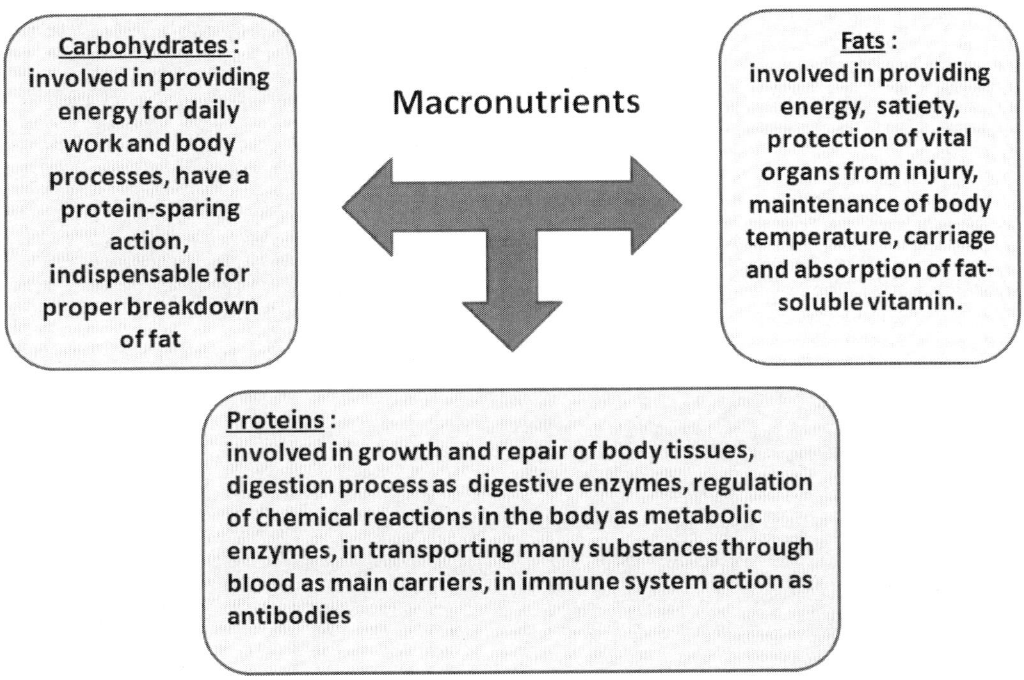

Figure 2. Macronutrients groups.

Even if total carbohydrate intake has not been related to periodontitis, the effect of dietary intake of some foods low in glycemic index (e.g. coarsely ground whole grain bread, beans and legumes, nuts, high-fiber fruits and vegetables) were also investigated. A large prospective study made on 34160 male US health professionals aged 40-75 yrs, showed that men in the highest quintile of whole-grain intake were 23% less likely to get periodontitis than were those in the lowest quintile (RR = 0.77; 95% CI: 0.66 - 0.89; $P<0.001$) after adjustment for age, smoking, body mass index, alcohol intake, physical activity, and total energy intake (Merchant et al, 2006). A new findings was that fruit consumption may play a protective role in periodontitis and to improve the periodontal therapy outcomes (Amaliya et al., 2015; Zare Javid et al., 2014; Jimenez et al., 2012; Chapple et al., 2012; Feghali K et al., 2011; Johansson et al., 1994; Blignaut & Grobler, 1992 ; Grobler & Blignaut, 1989).

Lipids are not so easily classified due to their many different structural features and chemical properties. The main categories are: 1) Simple Lipids (e.g. oils and fats); 2) Compound Lipids (e.g. Phospholipids, Glycolipids, Lipoproteins); 3) Derived Lipids (e.g. sterols and glycerol; carotenoids; and the fat-soluble vitamins A, D, E, and K).

It was revealed that a fat-enriched diet with a reduced amount of daily dietary fibers. known to induce inflammation-mediated insulin-resistance and glucose-intolerance (Riant et al, 2009), is also associated with a change in the intestinal microbiota ecology characterized by an increase in gram-negative bacteria (Turnbaugh et al., 2008; Turnbaugh et al., 2009) which is linked to the occurrence of type 2 diabetes. Moreover, several pathogenic gram negative bacteria are usually associated with the onset of periodontitis (Lakhssassi et al., 2005).

The diabetogenic fat-enriched diet induced in ovariectomised mice the increase of periodontal pathogenic microbiota like *Fusobacterium nucleatum* and *Prevotella intermedia* as well as the development of gingival inflammation and alveolar bone loss. These effects were prevented by chronic estrogen administration, as well as the deletion of CD14 (Blasco-Baque et al., 2012).

Fatty acids are the main building blocks of triglycerides and can be classified by the length of the carbon chain: 1) Saturated fatty acids; 2) Monounsaturated fatty acids (e.g. oleic acid also known as omega-9 found in olive oil, peanut oil, almonds, pecans, and avocados); and 3) Polyunsaturated fatty acids (PUFAs) (e.g. linoleic acid also known as omega-6 and alpha-linolenic acid also known as omega-3)(Tucker, 2010).

It has been showed that the omega-3 and omega-6 PUFAs showed strong antimicrobial activity against *Aggregatibacter segnis* KCTC 5968, *Fusobacterium nucleatum* subsp. *Polymorphum* KCTC 5172 and *Prevotella intermedia* KCTC 25611, and *Porphyromonas gingivalis* KCTC 381, all micro-organisms implicated in the etiology of gingivitis and periodontitis (Choi et al., 2013).

As anti-inflammatory properties have been reported for PUFAs, several studies have investigated their role in the modulation of gingival and periodontal disease indicating their potential therapeutic efficacy (Kesavalu et al., 2006; Naqvi et al., 2014; Araghizadeh et al., 2014; Choi et al., 2013; Figueredo et al., 2013; Raffaelli et al., 2008; Rosenstein et al., 2003; Eberhard et al., 2002; Campan et al., 1997).

6. Impact of Micronutrients on the Periodontal Disease Status

Micronutrients - are those nutrients required by the body in smaller amounts (Tucker, 2010) (Figure 3.).

Vitamin B-complex includes Vitamin B_1 (thiamine), Vitamin B_2 (riboflavin), (niacin or nicotinic acid), Vitamin B_5 (pantothenic acid), Vitamin B_6 (pyridoxine, pyridoxal, pyridoxamine), Vitamin B_7 (biotin), Vitamin B_9 (folic acid) and vitamin B_{12} (various cobalamins)(Singh, 2012). Staudte et al., (2012) highlighted that patients with periodontitis had significantly lower intake rates of folic acid than those of healthy controls, while Erdemir & Bergstrom (2006) revealed that among patients with periodontal disease the serum folic acid concentration is lower in smokers compared with non-smokers. Furthermore, vitamin-B complex can positively influence periodontal wound healing processes as vitamin B-complex supplement in combination with access flap surgery resulted in statistically significant superior clinical attachment level gains when compared to placebo (access flap surgery alone) in patients with generalized moderate to severe chronic periodontitis (Neiva et al., 2005).

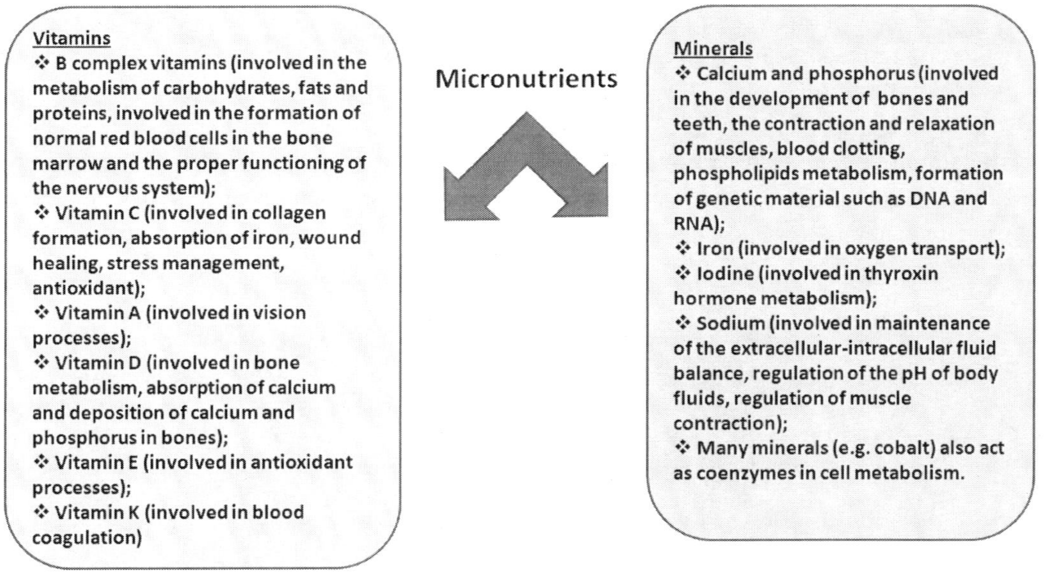

Figure 3. Micronutrients groups.

Vitamin C, or ascorbic acid, is a powerful antioxidant associated with absorption of iron, immunological functions (e.g. wound healing, phagocytosis) as well as in collagen formation in connective tissue such as the periodontium (**Figure 4.**).

Several recent studies indicate a relationship between plasma vitamin C and inflammation (Aguirre & May, 2008; Mohammed et al., 2014). *In vitro* models, vitamin C induces periodontal ligament progenitor cell differentiation, important for maintaining the homeostasis of PDL tissue and alveolar bone, via activation of ERK pathway mediated by PELP1 (Yan et al., 2013), partially antagonize the hydrogen peroxide-induced cytotoxicity in periodontal ligament cells (Wu et al., 2015) and attenuates the cytotoxic effects of Porphyromonas gingivalis on human gingival fibroblasts (Staudte et al., 2010).

In animal models, vitamin C attenuates the degree of experimental atherosclerosis induced by periodontitis in the rat by decreasing oxidative stress (Ekuni et al., 2009) and provides therapeutic effects on inhibition of alveolar bone resorption and periodontal tissue destruction (Akman et al., 2012) by down-regulating gene expression encoding inflammation, including interleukin-1 alpha and interleukin-1 beta (Tomofuji et al., 2009).

It is well known that smokers are almost three times more likely to have advanced periodontitis compared to the non-smokers (Johnson & Hill, 2004). Smoking is associated with alteration of antioxidant defenses, as well as upregulation of inflammation by a number of mechanisms leading to extensive oxidative damage and lower vitamin C levels were reported in smokers than in non-smokers (Palanisamy et al., 2009; Morrow et al., 1995) as well as in smokers with chronic periodontitis compared with non-smoker healthy controls and non-smokers with chronic periodontitis (Vit C in microM/l) : 22.7 ± 0.05 vs. 39.7 ± 0.06, respectively 28.3 ± 0.05) (Aziz et al., 2013).

The daily dietary intake of ascorbic acid may influence gingival bleeding level (Nishida et al., 2000; Leggott et al., 1986; Staudte et al., 2005; Gokhale et al., 2013). It has been showed that patients with periodontitis have a reduced intake of vitamin C (Staudte et al., 2012) and lower plasma vitamin C levels (Amaliya et al., 2007; Kuzmanova et al., 2012;

Thomas et al., 2010; Chapple et al., 2007; Amarasena et al., 2005; Pussinen et al., 2003) compared with healthy subjects. Moreover, single-nucleotide polymorphism rs6596473 in the vitamin C transporter SLC23A1 is associated with aggressive periodontitis (de Jong et al., 2014).

Vitamin C intake as an adjunct to conventional therapy such as scaling and root planing (SRP) yielded better results compared to SRP therapy alone significantly reduces the bleeding index (Gokhale et al., 2013) but also no adjunctive effect was reported (Abou Sulaiman et al., 2010), suggesting that further studies need to be performed in this field.

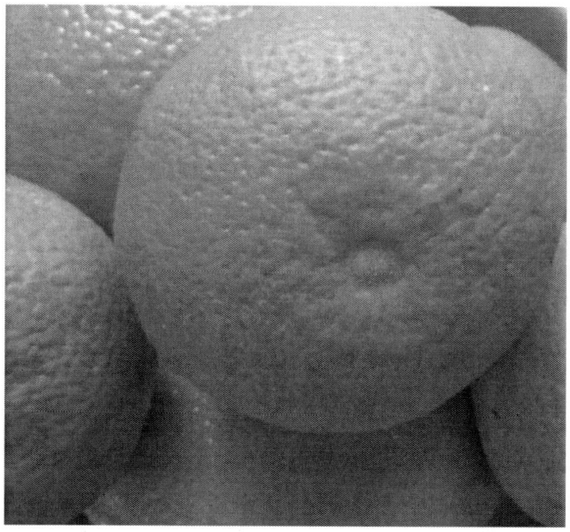

Figure 4. Oranges, like other citrus fruits, are an excellent source of vitamin C.

Vitamin A is a group of unsaturated nutritional organic compounds that includes retinol, retinal, retinoic acid, and several provitamin A carotenoids, among which beta-carotene is the most important. Alpha-carotene is found in root vegetables (e.g. carrots), beta-carotene sources are green leafy, root and fruiting vegetables, lycopene is found in fruiting vegetables (fresh tomato), lutein in green leafy vegetables, beta-cryptoxanthin in citrus fruits, citrus fruits and green leafy vegetables are the main source of zeaxanthin (García-Closas et al., 2004).

The positive use of vitamin A in periodontal diseases has yet to be evaluated in detail, even if it has been reported that:

- oral administration of all-trans retinoic acid has a potential for clinical prevention of periodontitis as it suppresses experimental periodontitis in mice by modulating the Th17/Treg imbalance (Wang et al., 2014);
- β-cryptoxanthin, a typical carotenoid, has also a protective effect against periodontal disease as in a mouse model of periodontitis, it suppressed bone resorption in the mandibular alveolar bone *in vitro* and restored alveolar bone loss induced by lipopolysaccharide (LPS) *in vivo* (Matsumoto et al., 2013). This preventive effect on bone resorption in periodontitis is modulated through inhibition of the production of IL-6 and IL-8 and up-regulation of osteoprotegerin (OPG) production (Nishigaki et al., 2013).

- Lycopene, a powerful antioxidant and the main carotenoid in tomato products is also been successfully used as an adjunct to scaling and root planing in gingivitis patients (Chandra et al., 2007), as an adjunct treatment modality to oral prophylaxis (full mouth scaling and root planing completed within 24 hours) in patients with moderate periodontal disease (Belludi et al., 2013) or as a gel formulation, effective in significant reductions in probing depths and gain in the clinical attachment levels compared with the placebo in smoking and nonsmoking subjects with chronic periodontitis (Chandra et al., 2012).

Vitamin D is essential for cell development, neuromuscular functioning, bone metabolism, absorption of calcium, deposition of calcium and phosphorus in bones bone development and inflammation control. As in periodontal inflammation, the alveolar bone re-absorption is a major characteristic, it was possible to consider that mediators of bone metabolism such as Vitamin D Receptor (VDR) and its genetic polymorphisms have an important a role in the individual susceptibility to developing periodontitis (Martelli et al., 2014). A recent meta-analysis investigated the association between vitamin D receptor polymorphisms (including four gene loci: *Taq-I*, *Bsm-I*, *Apa-I*, and *Fok-I*) for susceptibility to periodontitis. The results of the meta-analysis performed by Chen et al., (2012) on nineteen case-control studies concluded that "1) the mutant allele t of the *Taq-I* locus may be a protective factor for chronic but not for aggressive periodontitis in Asians, although this was not true in whites; 2) the mutant allele F of the *Fok-I* locus appeared to be a risk factor for aggressive rather than chronic periodontitis in Asians; and 3) *Bsm-I* and *Apa-I* polymorphisms were found to have no significant associations with susceptibility to periodontitis (chronic/aggressive)."

A significant relationship between serum and gingival crevicular fluid levels of vitamin D and periodontitis condition and/or tooth loss were reported by several studies (Antonoglou et al., 2015; Zhan et al., 2014; Zhang et al., 2014; Antonoglou et al., 2013; Bastos et al., 2013; Millen et al., 2013; Zhang et al., 2013; Zhou et al., 2012; Liu et al., 2010 ; Liu et al., 2009). Moreover, it was revealed not only an improving of the periodontal health after vitamin D intake in patients with periodontitis (Miley et al., 2009; Van der Velden et al., 2011; Garcia et al., 2011) but it was also suggested that vitamin D status may be critical for post-surgical healing (Bashutski et al., 2011).

Vitamin E refers to a group of compounds that include both tocopherols and tocotrienols mainly involved in antioxidant processes.

Carvalho et al., (2013) reported that vitamin E has the potential to reduce oxidative damage and inflammatory response in a ligature-induced periodontitis in rats but does not prevent alveolar bone loss. Clinical studies revealed controversial results with either failing to support the use of vitamin E as a topical chemotherapeutic agent for the control of gingivitis or periodontal disease (Slade et al., 1976; Cohen et al., 1991) either revealing that the adjunctive vitamin E supplementation improves periodontal healing (Asman et al., 1994; Singh et al., 2014).

Several studies have focused on the inter-relationship between various *minerals* and periodontal health status (Table 1.).

Table 1. Overview of clinical studies focused on the inter-relationship between various minerals and periodontal health status

Author, year	Minerals investigated	Main findings
Shimazaki et al., 2008	Calcium	The routine intake of lactic acid foods may have a beneficial effect on periodontal disease.
Nishida et al., 2000	Calcium	Low dietary intake of calcium results in more severe periodontal disease. The relationship between low dietary calcium intake and increased levels of periodontal disease showed an estimated odds ratio (OR) of 1.84 (95% CI: 1.36 to 2.48) for young males, 1.99 (95% CI: 1.34 to 2.97) for young females, and 1.90 (95% CI: 1.41 to 2.55) for the older group of males.
Ramesh et al., 2011	Calcium	Postmenopausal women exhibit a reduced alveolar bone mass and lowered levels of serum total calcium with the increasing age.
Amarasena et al., 2008	Calcium	Serum calcium may be considered a risk factor for periodontal disease progression in non-institutionalized elderly.
Kuraner et al., 1991	Calcium	Patients with periodontitis had increased Ca serum levels and decreased Ca levels in parotid saliva.
Kolte et al., 2012	Calcium and phosphorus	The present study exhibited reduced concentrations of, calcium and phosphorus in whole saliva in smokers with chronic periodontitis.
Muñoz et al., 2001	Calcium and phosphorus	Multi-vitamin nutritional supplement might be a beneficial adjunct to the required established periodontal treatment.
Thomas et al., 2013	Copper	The serum levels of copper increased in diabetes patients with periodontitis compared to healthy individuals with and without periodontitis.
Thomas et al., 2013	Iron	The serum levels of iron increased in diabetes patients with periodontitis compared to healthy individuals with and without periodontitis.
Rao et al., 2013	Iron	It has been concluded that periodontitis does not induce anemia like state, as the hematological and biochemical parameters were almost equally affected in periodontally healthy and periodontally diseased individuals.
Chakraborty et al., 2014	Iron	Iron deficiency anemia patients with chronic periodontitis have more periodontal breakdowns than patients with chronic periodontitis.
Prakash et al., 2012	Iron	The presence and severity of periodontitis may not affect the serum iron and serum ferritin parameters of an individual.
Pushparani et al., 2014	Magnesium	Patients with diabetes mellitus and periodontitis had altered metabolism of Zn and Mg.
Kolte et al., 2012	Magnesium	The present study exhibited reduced concentrations of magnesium in whole saliva in smokers with chronic periodontitis.
Staudte et al., 2012	Magnesium	Patients with periodontitis have a reduced intake of magnesium compared with healthy subjects.

Author, year	**Minerals investigated**	**Main findings**
Yoshihara et al., 2011	Magnesium	A low serum Ca/Mg ratio was significantly associated with periodontal disease progression in Japanese elderly smokers.
Meisel et al., 2005	Magnesium	Nutritional magnesium supplementation may improve periodontal health.
Tanaka et al., 2006	Magnesium	Intake of magnesium is related to reduced prevalence of tooth loss among young Japanese women.
Rodrigues et al., 2014	Phosphorus	In haemodialysis patients, the periodontitis group had phosphorus serum levels lower than the no periodontitis group.
Liu et al., 2009	Phosphorus	Serum inorganic phosphorus values of patients with chronic and aggressive periodontitis were lower than those of healthy controls.
Thomas et al., 2013	Selenium	The levels of selenium are significantly lower in diabetic patients with periodontitis and also in healthy individuals with periodontitis, but are highest in healthy controls, showing that the serum levels are inversely proportional to inflammation and tissue destruction.
Pushparani et al., 2014	Zinc	Patients with diabetes mellitus and periodontitis had altered metabolism of Zn and Mg.
Thomas et al., 2013	Zinc	The serum levels of zinc decreased in diabetes patients with periodontitis compared to healthy individuals with and without periodontitis.
Kuraner et al., 1991	Zinc	Patients with periodontitis had decreased Zn serum levels.

7. Impact of Dietary Excess on Periodontal Health

Over the past 30-40 years, changes in food composition and availability have contributed to the dramatic increase in obesity in developed and, increasingly, in developing countries (Morris et al., 2014). Unfortunately, this global obesity epidemic has been described by the World Health Organization as one of the most frequent but also one of the most neglected public health problems (Stevens et al., 2012) that is associated with frequent morbidities such as hypertension, angina, diabetes and arthritis (Shukla et al., 2014).

Both periodontal disease and obesity are among the most common chronic disorders affecting the world's populations, and several reviews suggest a potential link between **overweight/obesity** and periodontitis (Table 2.). Obesity appears to participate in the multifactorial phenomenon of causality of periodontitis, due to the abnormal or excessive deposition of fat in the adipose tissue that leads to a severe increase in oxidative stress, determining not only an endothelial dysfunction but also to the increase in proinflammatory cytokines, a negative effect that leads finally to periodontitis (Suresh et al., 2014; Boesing et al., 2009; Pischon et al., 2007).

Physical activity also independently reduces not only the risk of several general diseases (e.g. cardiac problems, diabetes, osteoporosis) but has been also associated with lower periodontitis prevalence, independent of obesity (Merchant et al., 2003; Al-Zahrani et al., 2005; Eberhard et al., 2014). Moreover, moderate and severe periodontitis were independently associated with low levels of high-sensitive C-reactive protein in sedentary men aged between 45 and 65 years (Sanders et al., 2009).

Table 2. Overview of Review Articles and Meta-Analyses focused on the inter-relationship between obesity and periodontal disease

Author, year	Type of Study	Main conclusion
Watanabe & Cho, 2014	Review	Metabolic syndrome is a conglomerate of several physical conditions/diseases that include glucose intolerance/insulin resistance, hypertension, obesity, and dyslipidemia. All the reviewed studies demonstrated a positive association between periodontal disease and metabolic syndrome.
Katz & Bimstein, 2011	Review	Further studies are needed to support the hypothesis that obesity in children may be associated with increased rates of periodontal disease.
Suvan et al., 2011	Meta-analyses	Meta-analyses indicated statistically significant associations between periodontitis and body mass index (BMI) category obese OR 1.81(1.42, 2.30), overweight OR 1.27(1.06, 1.51) and obese and overweight combined OR 2.13(1.40, 3.26).
Chaffee & Weston, 2010	Meta-analyses	A positive association was reported with a role for obesity in the development of periodontal disease. The fixed-effects summary odds ratio was 1.35 (Shore-corrected 95% confidence interval: 1.23 to 1.47), with some evidence of a stronger association found among younger adults, women, and non-smokers.
Keller et al., 2015	Review	This systematic review suggests that overweight, obesity, weight gain and increased waist circumference may be risk factors for development or worsening with regard to periodontal measures.

8. Impact of Caloric Restriction on Periodontal Health

Dietary caloric restriction has been found to reduce systemic markers of inflammation and to protect against age-associated diseases including chronic inflammatory disorders such as cardiovascular disease and diabetes (González et al., 2012; Ingram et al., 1990). Moreover, several studies on animal models revealed that long-term caloric restriction has a significant impact on reducing the extent and severity of naturally occurring chronic periodontal disease, local inflammatory and immune responses, and periodontal microbiology (Reynolds et al., 2009; Branch-Mays et al., 2008).

Undernutrition is defined as a disturbance of form or function arising from the deficiency of one or more nutrients. Undernutrition can be classified as being mild or severe, helpful (if it results in appropriate weight loss in someone who is obese), or dangerous. Weight loss is associated not only with fat lost from adipose tissue but also with depletion of essential nutrients, protein (apparent in two main ways: somatic protein depletion, e.g. loss of muscular tissue, and visceral protein depletion, e.g. protein loss from the liver, pancreas and gut) and micronutrients (Schenker, 2003).

Malnutrition-Inflammation Complex Syndrome (MICS) or **Malnutrition-inflammation atherosclerosis** refers to the co-morbidity of protein-energy malnutrition and inflammation that oare highly prevalent in maintenance haemodialysis patients. MICS is associated with a poor outcome, including a decreased quality of life, refractory anaemia and significantly greater rates of hospitalization and mortality (Anand et al., 2013). The periodontal health is frequently in poor condition in haemodialysis patients and the periodontal status often correlates with the markers of malnutrition and inflammation (Strippoli et al., 2013; Chen et al., 2006).

9. Impact of Alcohol Use/Abuse on Periodontal Health

Alcohol consumption in higher amounts and on a long-term basis can determine a toxic damage of the organism through a manipulation of the host defenses causing a wide variety of diseases such as oral and oropharyngeal cancer (Huber & Tantiwongkosi, 2014), esophageal cancer(Franke et al., 2005), laryngeal cancer (Coca-Pelaz et al., 2013), gastric cancer (Massarrat & Stolte, 2014), liver cirrhosis (Louvet & Mathurin, 2015), pancreatitis (Muniraj et al., 2014), cardiovascular problems (Notara et al., 2014), obesity (Traversy & Chaput, 2015), diabetes (Kim et al., 2015), stroke (Senoo et al., 2014), and even mental disorders (e.g. depression) (Gea et al., 2013).

A recent systematic review, performed by Amaral et al., (2009), has evaluated the studies focused on the relationship between alcohol dependence/consumption and periodontal disease. The research was comprehensive and included several databases such as PUBMED Medline, Latin American and Caribean Health Science-LILACS, Scientific electronic library online-SciELO and Cochrane Central Register of Controlled Trials-CCRT literature databases from January 1965 to July 2008. Of the 1530 papers identified, only 11 cross-sectional and 5 longitudinal observational studies met the inclusion criteria. No meta-analysis was performed due to the high heterogeneity among studies concerning the methods of assessment of alcohol dependence, alcohol consumption and periodontitis (Amaral et al., 2009).

Moreover, the confounding effect of dental plaque was taken into account in only 6 studies. Based on the fact that seven of the twelve articles on alcohol consumption and 4 of the 4 studies on alcohol dependence reported positive associations between alcohol intake and periodontitis, Amaral et al., (2009) concluded that alcohol consumption can be considered a risk indicator for periodontitis.

10. Proposed Mechanisms of How Diet May Impact on the Periodontal Tissues

The mechanisms by which dietary factors affect inflammatory processes at a cellular and molecular level were elucidated and presented by Chapple (2009) and by Milward & Chapple (2015).

The periodontitis phenotype is characterized by hyperinflammation. Oxidative stress has been proposed as a potential mechanistic link between periodontitis and systemic disease. Increased levels of oxidative stress can be triggered not only from cellular metabolism or from the host's response to periodontal pathogenic bacteria such as *Porphyromonas gingivalis* but also by the increased dietary intake of simple sugars or saturated fat by receptor binding of neutrophils.

As a consequence, the levels of oxidative stress and the periodontal inflammatory sequelae can be reduced by two modalities: 1) by the reduction of dietary refined carbohydrates and saturated fats and 2) by the increase diet rich in antioxidants and specific micronutrients. Examples of foods rich in antioxidants are green leafy vegetables, red beans, red wine, berries and dark chocolate with greater than 70% cocoa (Chapple, 2009; Milward & Chapple, 2015).

11. Tooth Loss and Its Impact on Dietary Intake

Advanced periodontal disease is leads to alveolar bone resorption and finally to tooth loss. One of the most immediate and important functional consequences of edentulous tooth loss is a reduction in chewing ability and masticatory ability, as well as several non-dental functional impairments, such as decreased biting force and reduced saliva flow (Ono et al., 2003; Peyron et al., 2004; Shinkawa et al., 2009; Kim et al., 2009).

When the ability to chew foods is compromised by the oral health status, having few or no natural teeth, the individuals begin to select a diet that they can chew in comfort. Generally, there is not only a change in food's choice (a diet low in fruits and vegetables intake and reduced in both non-starch polysaccharide and micronutrient intakes) but also a trend for reduced dietary intake overall (Samnieng et al., 2011; Walls & Steele, 2004). Moreover, reduced salivary flow and function may affect also the individuals' ability to chew and swallow (Walls & Steele, 2004). Finally these nutritional problems will affect the general health, the psychological and social well-being as well as the life quality (Nguyen et al., 2011; Brennan et al., 2008).

12. Dietary Recommendations for Periodontal Disease Management

As the periodontal scientific community is starting to understand the health benefits of diets rich in antioxidants and omega-3 polyunsaturated fatty acids, as well as the high problems of diets high in refined carbohydrates, the 2011 European workshop on Periodontology (Chapple et al., 2012) recommended that:

> *"the dental team should consider including advice to all patients on increasing levels of fish oils, fiber, fruit and vegetables and to reduce levels of refined sugars as part of a periodontal prevention/treatment regime and a general health benefit message."*

References

Abiko Y, Shimono M. Regeneration of periodontal tissues following experimentally induced periodontitis in rats: a comparison of sucrose-rich and conventional diets. *Bull Tokyo Dent Coll.* 1989;30(4):195-204.

Abou Sulaiman AE, Shehadeh RM. Assessment of total antioxidant capacity and the use of vitamin C in the treatment of non-smokers with chronic periodontitis. *J. Periodontol.* 2010;81(11):1547-54.

Aguirre R, May JM. Inflammation in the vascular bed: importance of vitamin C. *Pharmacol Ther.* 2008;119(1):96-103.

Akman S, Canakci V, Kara A, Tozoglu U, Arabaci T, Dagsuyu IM. Therapeutic effects of alpha lipoic acid and vitamin C on alveolar bone resorption after experimental periodontitis in rats: a biochemical, histochemical, and stereologic study. *J. Periodontol.* 2013;84(5):666-74.

Al-Zahrani MS, Borawski EA, Bissada NF. Increased physical activity reduces prevalence of periodontitis. *J. Dent.* 2005;33(9):703-10.

Amaliya, Laine ML, Delanghe JR, Loos BG, Van Wijk AJ, Van der Velden U. Java project on periodontal diseases. Periodontal bone loss in relation to environmental and systemic conditions. *J. Clin Periodontol.* 2015;42:325-332.

Amaliya, Timmerman MF, Abbas F, Loos BG, Van der Weijden GA, Van Winkelhoff AJ, Winkel EG, Van der Velden U. Java project on periodontal diseases: the relationship between vitamin C and the severity of periodontitis. *J. Clin. Periodontol.* 2007;34(4):299-304.

Amaral Cda S, Vettore MV, Leão A. The relationship of alcohol dependence and alcohol consumption with periodontitis: a systematic review. *J. Dent.* 2009;37(9):643-51.

Amarasena N, Ogawa H, Yoshihara A, Hanada N, Miyazaki H. Serum vitamin C-periodontal relationship in community-dwelling elderly Japanese. *J. Clin. Periodontol.* 2005;32(1):93-7.

Amarasena N, Yoshihara A, Hirotomi T, Takano N, Miyazaki H. Association between serum calcium and periodontal disease progression in non-institutionalized elderly. *Gerodontology.* 2008;25(4):245-50.

Anand N, S C C, Alam MN. The malnutrition inflammation complex syndrome-the micsing factor in the perio-chronic kidney disease interlink. *J. Clin. Diagn. Res.* 2013;7(4):763-7.

Antonoglou G, Knuuttila M, Niemelä O, Hiltunen L, Raunio T, Karttunen R, Vainio O, Ylöstalo P, Tervonen T. Serum 1,25(OH)D level increases after elimination of periodontal inflammation in T1DM subjects. *J. Clin. Endocrinol Metab.* 2013;98(10):3999-4005.

Antonoglou GN, Knuuttila M, Niemelä O, Raunio T, Karttunen R, Vainio O, Hedberg P, Ylöstalo P, Tervonen T. Low serum level of 1,25(OH)2 D is associated with chronic periodontitis. *J. Periodontal. Res.* 2015;50(2):274-80.

Araghizadeh N, Paknejad M, Alaeddini M, Minaii B, Abdollahi M, Khorasanie R. The efficacy and prophylactic characteristics of omega-3 fatty acids in experimental gingivitis in rats. *Iran J. Basic Med. Sci.* 2014;17(2):87-92.

Asman B, Wijkander P, Hjerpe A. Reduction of collagen degradation in experimental gingival tissue by vitamin E and Selenium. *J. Clin. Periodontol.* 1994;21:45.

Aziz AS, Kalekar MG, Suryakar AN, Benjamin T, Prakashan MJ, Ahmed BM, Sayyad M. Assessment of some biochemical oxidative stress markers in male smokers with chronic periodontitis. *Indian J. Clin. Biochem.* 2013;28(4):374-80.

Baer PN, Hawkins GR, Wells H, Mantel N, Zipkin I. Studies on experimental calculus formation in the rat. XI. Relation to diet and selected salivary constituents. *J. Periodontol.* 1967;38(4):323-9.

Bashutski JD, Eber RM, Kinney JS, Benavides E, Maitra S, Braun TM, Giannobile WV, McCauley LK. The impact of vitamin D status on periodontal surgery outcomes. *J. Dent. Res.* 2011;90(8):1007-12.

Bastos Jdo A, Andrade LC, Ferreira AP, Barroso Ede A, Daibert Pde C, Barreto PL, Vilela EM, Marcaccini AM, Colugnati FA, Bastos MG. [Serum levels of vitamin D and chronic periodontitis in patients with chronic kidney disease]. *J. Bras. Nefrol.* 2013;35(1):20-6.

Baumgartner S, Imfeld T, Schicht O, Rath C, Persson RE, Persson GR. The impact of the stone age diet on gingival conditions in the absence of oral hygiene. *J. Periodontol.* 2009;80(5):759-68.

Beauman C, Cannon G, Elmadfa I, Glasauer P, Hoffmann I, Keller M, Krawinkel M,Lang T, Leitzmann C, Lötsch B, Margetts BM, McMichael AJ, Meyer-Abich K,Oltersdorf U, Pettoello-Mantovani M, Sabaté J, Shetty P, Sória M, Spiekermann U, Tudge C, Vorster HH, Wahlqvist M, Zerilli-Marimò M. The principles, definition and dimensions of the new nutrition science. *Public Health Nutr.* 2005;8(6A):695-8.

Beers, Mark H, MD, Robert Berkow, MD, editors. ''Malnutrition.'' Section 1, Chapter 2. In The Merck manual of diagnosis and therapy. Whitehouse Station, NJ: Merck Research Laboratories, 2004.

Belludi SA, Verma S, Banthia R, Bhusari P, Parwani S, Kedia S, Saiprasad SV. Effect of lycopene in the treatment of periodontal disease: a clinical study. *J. Contemp. Dent. Pract.* 2013;14(6):1054-9.

Björnsson MJ, Velschow S, Stoltze K, Havemose-Poulsen A, Schou S, Holmstrup P. The influence of diet consistence, drinking water and bedding on periodontal disease in Sprague-Dawley rats. *J. Periodontal. Res.* 2003;38(6):543-50.

Blasco-Baque V, Serino M, Vergnes JN, Riant E, Loubieres P, Arnal JF, Gourdy P, Sixou M, Burcelin R, Kemoun P. High-fat diet induces periodontitis in mice through lipopolysaccharides (LPS) receptor signaling: protective action of estrogens. *PLoS One.* 2012;7(11):e48220.

Blignaut JB, Grobler SR. High fruit consumption and the periodontal status of farm workers. *Clin. Prev. Dent.* 1992;14(2):25-8.

Boesing F, Patiño JS, da Silva VR, Moreira EA. The interface between obesity and periodontitis with emphasis on oxidative stress and inflammatory response. *Obes. Rev.* 2009;10(3):290-7.

Boyd LD, Lampi KJ. Importance of nutrition for optimum health of the periodontium. *J. Contemp. Dent. Pract.* 2001;2(2):36-45.

Boyd LD, Madden TE. Nutrition, infection, and periodontal disease. *Dent. Clin. N. Am.* 2003;47(2):337-54.

Branch-Mays GL, Dawson DR, Gunsolley JC, Reynolds MA, Ebersole JL, Novak KF, Mattison JA, Ingram DK, Novak MJ. The effects of a calorie-reduced diet on periodontal inflammation and disease in a non-human primate model. *J. Periodontol.* 2008;79(7):1184-91.

Brennan DS, Spencer AJ, Roberts-Thomson KF. Tooth loss, chewing ability and quality of life. *Qual Life Res.* 2008;17(2):227-35.

Bsoul SA, Terezhalmy GT. Vitamin C in health and disease. *J. Contemp. Dent. Pract* 2004;5(2):1-13.

Campan P, Planchand PO, Duran D. Pilot study on n-3 polyunsaturated fatty acids in the treatment of human experimental gingivitis. *J. Clin. Periodontol.* 1997;24(12):907-13.

Cannon G, Leitzmann C. The new nutrition science project. *Public Health Nutr.* 2005;8(6A):673-94.

Carvalho Rde S, de Souza CM, Neves JC, Holanda-Pinto SA, Pinto LM, Brito GA, de Andrade GM. Vitamin E does not prevent bone loss and induced anxiety in rats with ligature-induced periodontitis. *Arch. Oral Biol.* 2013;58(1):50-8.

Chaffee BW, Weston SJ. Association between chronic periodontal disease and obesity: a systematic review and meta-analysis. *J. Periodontol.* 2010;81(12):1708-24.

Chakraborty S, Tewari S, Sharma RK, Narula SC, Ghalaut PS, Ghalaut V. Impact of iron deficiency anemia on chronic periodontitis and superoxide dismutase activity: a cross-sectional study. *J. Periodontal. Implant. Sci.* 2014;44(2):57-64.

Chandra RV, Prabhuji ML, Roopa DA, Ravirajan S, Kishore HC. Efficacy of lycopene in the treatment of gingivitis: a randomised, placebo-controlled clinical trial. *Oral Health Prev. Dent.* 2007;5(4):327-36.

Chandra RV, Sandhya YP, Nagarajan S, Reddy BH, Naveen A, Murthy KR. Efficacy of lycopene as a locally delivered gel in the treatment of chronic periodontitis: smokers vs nonsmokers. *Quintessence Int.* 2012;43(5):401-11.

Chapple IL, Milward MR, Dietrich T. The prevalence of inflammatory periodontitis is negatively associated with serum antioxidant concentrations. *J. Nutr.* 2007 Mar;137(3):657-64.

Chapple IL, Milward MR, Ling-Mountford N, Weston P, Carter K, Askey K, Dallal GE, De Spirt S, Sies H, Patel D, Matthews JB. Adjunctive daily supplementation with encapsulated fruit, vegetable and berry juice powder concentrates and clinical periodontal outcomes: a double-blind RCT. *J. Clin. Periodontol.* 2012;39(1):62-72.

Chapple IL. Potential mechanisms underpinning the nutritional modulation of periodontal inflammation. *J. Am. Dent. Assoc.* 2009;140(2):178-84.

Chen LP, Chiang CK, Chan CP, Hung KY, Huang CS. Does periodontitis reflect inflammation and malnutrition status in hemodialysis patients? *Am. J. Kidney Dis.* 2006;47(5):815-22.

Choi JS, Park NH, Hwang SY, Sohn JH, Kwak I, Cho KK, Choi IS. The antibacterial activity of various saturated and unsaturated fatty acids against several oral pathogens. *J. Environ. Biol.* 2013;34(4):673-6.

Coca-Pelaz A, Rodrigo JP, Takes RP, Silver CE, Paccagnella D, Rinaldo A, Hinni ML, Ferlito A. Relationship between reflux and laryngeal cancer. *Head Neck.* 2013;35(12):1814-8.

Cohen RE, Ciancio SG, Mather ML, Curro FA. Effect of vitamin E gel, placebo gel and chlorhexidine on periodontal disease. *Clin. Prev. Dent.* 1991;13(5):20-4.

Crawford JM, Taubman MA, Smith DJ. The natural history of periodontal bone loss in germfree and gnotobiotic rats infected with periodontopathic microorganisms. *J. Periodontal. Res.* 1978;13(4):316-25.

de Jong TM, Jochens A, Jockel-Schneider Y, Harks I, Dommisch H, Graetz C, Flachsbart F, Staufenbiel I, Eberhard J, Folwaczny M, Noack B, Meyle J, Eickholz P, Gieger C, Grallert H, Lieb W, Franke A, Nebel A, Schreiber S, Doerfer C, Jepsen S, Bruckmann C, van der Velden U, Loos BG, Schaefer AS. SLC23A1 polymorphism rs6596473 in the vitamin C transporter SVCT1 is associated with aggressive periodontitis. *J. Clin. Periodontol.* 2014;41(6):531-40.

Dorsky R. Nutrition and oral health. *Gen. Dent.* 2001;49(6):576-82.

Eberhard J, Heilmann F, Açil Y, Albers HK, Jepsen S. Local application of n-3 or n-6 polyunsaturated fatty acids in the treatment of human experimental gingivitis. *J. Clin. Periodontol.* 2002;29(4):364-9.

Eberhard J, Stiesch M, Kerling A, Bara C, Eulert C, Hilfiker-Kleiner D, Hilfiker A, Budde E, Bauersachs J, Kück M, Haverich A, Melk A, Tegtbur U. Moderate and severe periodontitis are independent risk factors associated with low cardiorespiratory fitness in sedentary non-smoking men aged between 45 and 65 years. *J. Clin. Periodontol.* 2014;41(1):31-7.

Ekuni D, Tomofuji T, Sanbe T, Irie K, Azuma T, Maruyama T, Tamaki N, Murakami J, Kokeguchi S, Yamamoto T. Vitamin C intake attenuates the degree of experimental atherosclerosis induced by periodontitis in the rat by decreasing oxidative stress. *Arch. Oral Biol.* 2009;54(5):495-502.

Enwonwu CO, Phillips RS, Falkler WA Jr. Nutrition and oral infectious diseases: state of the science. *Compend. Contin. Educ. Dent.* 2002;23(5):431-4, 436, 438 passim; quiz 448.

Enwonwu CO, Phillips RS, Ibrahim CD, Danfillo IS. Nutrition and oral health in Africa. *Int. Dent. J.* 2004;54(6Suppl 1):344-51.

Enwonwu CO, Ritchie CS. Nutrition and inflammatory markers. *J. Am. Dent. Assoc.* (1939) 2007;138(1):70-73.

Enwonwu CO. Cellular and molecular effects of malnutrition and their relevance to periodontal diseases. *J. Clin. Periodontol* 1994;21(10):643-57.

Enwonwu CO. Interference of malnutrition and periodontal diseases. *Am. J. Clin. Nutr* 1995;6;430S-436S.

Erdemir EO, Bergstrom J. Relationship between smoking and folic acid, vitamin B12 and some haematological variables in patients with chronic periodontal disease. *J. Clin. Periodontol.* 2006;33(12):878-84.

EUFIC. Food-Based Dietary Guidelines in Europe 2009.Retrieved on 18 March 2015 on http://www.eufic.org/article/en/expid/food

Feghali K, Feldman M, La VD, Santos J, Grenier D. Cranberry proanthocyanidins: natural weapons against periodontal diseases. *J. Agric. Food* 2012;60(23):5728-35.

Figueredo CM, Martinez GL, Koury JC, Fischer RG, Gustafsson A. Serum levels of long-chain polyunsaturated fatty acids in patients with periodontal disease. *J. Periodontol.* 2013;84(5):675-82.

Franke A, Teyssen S, Singer MV. Alcohol-related diseases of the esophagus and stomach. *Dig. Dis.* 2005;23(3-4):204-13.

Garant PR, Cho MI. Histopathogenesis of spontaneous periodontal disease in conventional rats. III. The mononuclear cell infiltrate and cytoplasmic changes in associated fibroblasts. *J. Periodontal. Res.* 1980;15(2):165-76.

Garant PR, Cho MI. Histopathogenesis of spontaneous periodontal disease in conventional rats. I. Histometric and histologic study. *J. Periodontal. Res.* 1979;14(4):297-309.

Garcia MN, Hildebolt CF, Miley DD, Dixon DA, Couture RA, Spearie CL, Langenwalter EM, Shannon WD, Deych E, Mueller C, Civitelli R. One-year effects of vitamin D and calcium supplementation on chronic periodontitis. *J. Periodontol.* 2011;82(1):25-32.

Gea A, Beunza JJ, Estruch R, Sánchez-Villegas A, Salas-Salvadó J, Buil-Cosiales P, Gómez-Gracia E, Covas MI, Corella D, Fiol M, Arós F, Lapetra J, Lamuela-Raventós RM, Wärnberg J, Pintó X, Serra-Majem L, Martínez-González MA; PREDIMED GROUP. Alcohol intake, wine consumption and the development of depression: the PREDIMED study. *BMC Med.* 2013;11:192.

Gokhale NH, Acharya AB, Patil VS, Trivedi DJ, Thakur SL. A short-term evaluation of the relationship between plasma ascorbic acid levels and periodontal disease in systemically healthy and type 2 diabetes mellitus subjects. *J. Diet Suppl.* 2013;10(2):93-104.

González O, Tobia C, Ebersole J, Novak MJ. Caloric restriction and chronic inflammatory diseases. *Oral Dis.* 2012;18(1):16-31.

Grobler SR, Blignaut JB. The effect of a high consumption of apples or grapes on dental caries and periodontal disease in humans. *Clin. Prev. Dent.* 1989;11(1):8-12.

Heijl L, Wennström J, Lindhe J, Socransky SS. Periodontal disease in gnotobiotic rats. *J. Periodontal Res.* 1980;15(4):405-19.

Hornick B. Diet and nutrition implications for oral health. *J. Dent. Hyg.* 2002 Winter;76(1):67-78; quiz 79-81.

Huber MA, Tantiwongkosi B. Oral and oropharyngeal cancer. *Med. Clin. North Am.* 2014;98(6):1299-321.

Ingram DK, Cutler RG, Weindruch R, Renquist DM, Knapka JJ, April M, Belcher CT, Clark MA, Hatcherson CD, Marriott BM, et al., Dietary restriction and aging: the initiation of a primate study. *J. Gerontol.* 1990;45(5):B148-63.

Jimenez M, Hu FB, Marino M, Li Y, Joshipura KJ. Type 2 diabetes mellitus and 20 year incidence of periodontitis and tooth loss. *Diabetes Res. Clin. Pract.* 2012;98(3):494-500.

Johansson I, Tidehag P, Lundberg V, Hallmans G. Dental status, diet and cardiovascular risk factors in middle-aged people in northern Sweden. *Community Dent Oral Epidemiol.* 1994;22(6):431-6.

Johnson GK, Hill M. Cigarette smoking and the periodontal patient. *J. Periodontol.* 2004;75:196–209.

Johnson NW, Curtis MA. Preventive therapy for periodontal diseases. *Adv. Dent. Res.* 1994;8(2):337-48.

Karp WB. Nutrition update for the dental health professional. J. Calif. Dent. Assoc 1994;22(8):26-9.

Katz J, Bimstein E. Pediatric obesity and periodontal disease: a systematic review of the literature. *Quintessence Int.* 2011;42(7):595-9.

Keller A, Rohde JF, Raymond K, Heitmann BL. The Association Between Periodontal Disease and Overweight and Obesity: A Systematic Review. *J. Periodontol.* 2015;12:1-15.

Kesavalu L, Vasudevan B, Raghu B, Browning E, Dawson D, Novak JM, Correll MC, Steffen MJ, Bhattacharya A, Fernandes G, Ebersole JL. Omega-3 fatty acid effect on alveolar bone loss in rats. *J. Dent Res.* 2006;85(7):648-52.

Kim BI, Jeong SH, Chung KH, Cho YK, Kwon HK, Choi CH. Subjective food intake ability in relation to maximal bite force among Korean adults. *J. Oral Rehabil.* 2009;36(3):168-75.

Kim JY, Lee DY, Lee YJ, Park KJ, Kim KH, Kim JW, Kim WH. Chronic alcohol consumption potentiates the development of diabetes through pancreatic β-cell dysfunction. *World J. Biol. Chem.* 2015;6(1):1-15.

Kolte AP, Kolte RA, Laddha RK. Effect of smoking on salivary composition and periodontal status. *J. Indian Soc. Periodontol.* 2012;16(3):350-3.

Kulkarni V, Bhatavadekar NB, Uttamani JR. The effect of nutrition on periodontal disease: a systematic review. *J. Calif. Dent. Assoc.* 2014;42(5):302-11.

Kuraner T, Beksac MS, Kayakirilmaz K, Cağlayan F, Onderoğlu LS, Ozgünes H. Serum and parotid saliva testosterone, calcium, magnesium, and zinc levels in males, with and without periodontitis. *Biol. Trace Elem. Res.* 1991;31(1):43-9.

Kuzmanova D, Jansen ID, Schoenmaker T, Nazmi K, Teeuw WJ, Bizzarro S, Loos BG, van der Velden U. Vitamin C in plasma and leucocytes in relation to periodontitis. *J. Clin. Periodontol.* 2012;39(10):905-12.

Lakhssassi N, Elhajoui N, Lodter JP, Pineill JL, Sixou M. Antimicrobial susceptibility variation of 50 anaerobic periopathogens in aggressive periodontitis: an interindividual variability study. *Oral Microbiol. Immunol.* 2005;20(4):244-52.

Leggott PJ, Robertson PB, Rothman DL, Murray PA, Jacob RA. The eff ect of controlled ascorbic acid depletion and supplementation on periodontal health. *J. Periodontol.* 1986;57(8):480-5.

Leitzmann C, Cannon G. Dimensions, domains and principles of the new nutrition science. *Public Health Nutr.* 2005;8(6A):787-94.

Lekic P, Klausen B, Friis-Hasche E, Beloica D, Knezevic M, Hougen HP. Influence of age and immunization on development of gingivitis in rats. *Acta Odontol Scand.* 1989;47:233–8.

Liu K, Meng H, Lu R, Xu L, Zhang L, Chen Z, Shi D, Feng X, Tang X. Initial periodontal therapy reduced systemic and local 25-hydroxy vitamin D(3) and interleukin-1beta in patients with aggressive periodontitis. *J. Periodontol.* 2010;81(2):260-6.

Liu K, Meng H, Tang X, Xu L, Zhang L, Chen Z, Shi D, Feng X, Lu R. Elevated plasma calcifediol is associated with aggressive periodontitis. *J. Periodontol.* 2009;80(7):1114-20.

Louvet A, Mathurin P. Alcoholic liver disease: mechanisms of injury and targeted treatment. *Nat. Rev. Gastroenterol. Hepatol.* 2015;12(4):231-242.

Martelli FS, Martelli M, Rosati C, Fanti E. Vitamin D: relevance in dental practice. *Clin. Cases Miner Bone Metab*. 2014;11(1):15-9.

Massarrat S, Stolte M. Development of gastric cancer and its prevention. *Arch. Iran Med.* 2014;17(7):514-20.

Matsumoto C, Ashida N, Yokoyama S, Tominari T, Hirata M, Ogawa K, Sugiura M, Yano M, Inada M, Miyaura C. The protective effects of β-cryptoxanthin on inflammatory bone resorption in a mouse experimental model of periodontitis. *Biosci. Biotechnol. Biochem.* 2013;77(4):860-2.

Meisel P, Schwahn C, Luedemann J, John U, Kroemer HK, Kocher T. Magnesium deficiency is associated with periodontal disease. *J. Dent. Res.* 2005;84(10):937-41.

Merchant AT, Pitiphat W, Franz M, Joshipura KJ. Whole-grain and fiber intakes and periodontitis risk in men. *Am. J. Clin. Nutr.* 2006;83(6):1395-400.

Merchant AT, Pitiphat W, Rimm EB, Joshipura K. Increased physical activity decreases periodontitis risk in men. *Eur. J. Epidemiol.* 2003;18(9):891-8.

Miley DD, Garcia MN, Hildebolt CF, Shannon WD, Couture RA, Anderson Spearie CL, et al., Cross-sectional Study of Vitamin D and Calcium Supplementation Effects on Chronic Periodontitis. *J. Periodontol.* 2009;80(9):1433-1439.

Millen AE, Hovey KM, LaMonte MJ, Swanson M, Andrews CA, Kluczynski MA, Genco RJ, Wactawski-Wende J. Plasma 25-hydroxyvitamin D concentrations and periodontal disease in postmenopausal women. *J. Periodontol.* 2013;84(9):1243-56.

Milward MR, Chapple ILC. The role of diet in periodontal disease. Retrieved on March 23, 2015 on *www.bsdht.org.uk/res/DH%20May%20p18-21.pdf*

Mohammed BM, Fisher BJ, Huynh QK, Wijesinghe DS, Chalfant CE, Brophy DF, Fowler AA 3rd, Natarajan R. Resolution of sterile inflammation: role for vitamin C. *Mediators Inflamm.* 2014;2014:173403.

Morris MJ, Beilharz JE, ManiAm. J., Reichelt AC, Westbrook RF. Why is obesity such a problem in the 21st century? The intersection of palatable food, cues and reward pathways, stress, and cognition. *Neurosci Biobehav Rev*. 2014;pii:S0149-7634(14)00333-9.

Morrow JD, Balz F, Longmaire AW, Gaziamo JM, Lynch SM, Shyr Y, Strauss WE, Oates JA, Roberts LJ. Increase in circulatory products of lipid peroxidation (F_2-isoprostanes) in smokers. *N. Engl. J. Med.* 1995;332:1198–1203.

Muniraj T, Aslanian HR, Farrell J, Jamidar PA. Chronic pancreatitis, a comprehensive review and update. Part I: epidemiology, etiology, risk factors, genetics, pathophysiology, and clinical features. *Dis. Mon.* 2014;60(12):530-50.

Muñoz CA, Kiger RD, Stephens JA, Kim J, Wilson AC. Effects of a nutritional supplement on periodontal status. *Compend. Contin. Educ. Dent* .2001;22(5):425-8, 430, 432 passim; quiz 440.

Naqvi AZ, Hasturk H, Mu L, Phillips RS, Davis RB, Halem S, Campos H, Goodson JM, Van Dyke TE, Mukamal KJ. Docosahexaenoic Acid and Periodontitis in Adults: *A Randomized Controlled Trial. J. Dent. Res.* 2014 Jun 26;93(8):767-773.

Neiva RF, Al-Shammari K, Nociti FH Jr, Soehren S, Wang HL. Effects of vitamin-B complex supplementation on periodontal wound healing. *J. Periodontol.* 2005;76(7):1084-91.

Neiva RF, Steigenga J, Al-Shammari KF, Wang HL. Effects of specifi c nutrients on periodontal disease onset, progression and treatment. *J. Clin. Periodontol.* 2003;30(7):579-589.

Nguyen TC, Witter DJ, Bronkhorst EM, Gerritsen AE, Creugers NH. Chewing ability and dental functional status. *Int. J. Prosthodont.* 2011;24(5):428-36.

Nishida M, Grossi SG, Dunford RG, Ho AW, Trevisan M, Genco RJ. Calcium and the risk for periodontal disease. *J. Periodontol.* 2000;71(7):1057-1066.

Nishida M, Grossi SG, Dunford RG, Ho AW, Trevisan M, Genco RJ. Dietary vitamin C and the risk for periodontal disease. *J. Periodontol.* 2000;71(8):1215-23.

Nishigaki M, Yamamoto T, Ichioka H, Honjo K, Yamamoto K, Oseko F, Kita M, Mazda O, Kanamura N. β-cryptoxanthin regulates bone resorption related-cytokine production in human periodontal ligament cells. *Arch. Oral Biol.* 2013;58(7):880-6.

Notara V, Panagiotakos DB, Pitsavos CE. Secondary prevention of acute coronary syndrome. Socio-economic and lifestyle determinants: a literature review. *Cent Eur. J. Public Health.* 2014;22(3):175-82.

Ono T, Hori K, Ikebe K, Nokubi T, Nago S, Kumakura I. Factors influencing eating ability of old in-patients in a rehabilitation hospital in Japan. Gerodontology. 2003;20(1):24-31.

Palanisamy P, Rao YY, Farook J, Saravanan G, Bakthavathsalam G. Effect of cigarette smoking on lipids and oxidative stress biomarkers in patients with acute myocardial infarction. *Res. J. Med. Med. Sci.* 2009;4(2):151–159.

Peyron MA, Blanc O, Lund JP, Woda A. Influence of age on adaptability of human mastication. *J. Neurophysiol.* 2004;92(2):773-9.

Pischon N, Heng N, Bernimoulin JP, Kleber BM, Willich SN, Pischon T. Obesity, inflammation, and periodontal disease. *J. Dent. Res.* 2007;86(5):400-9.

Prakash S, Dhingra K, Priya S. Similar hematological and biochemical parameters among periodontitis and control group subjects. *Eur. J. Dent.* 2012;6(3):287-94.

Pushparani DS, Anandan SN, Theagarayan P. Serum zinc and magnesium concentrations in type 2 diabetes mellitus with periodontitis. *J. Indian Soc. Periodontol.* 2014;18(2):187-93.

Pussinen PJ, Laatikainen T, Alfthan G, Asikainen S, Jousilahti P. Periodontitis is associated with a low concentration of vitamin C in plasma. *Clin. Diagn. Lab. Immunol.* 2003;10(5):897-902.

Raffaelli L, Serini S, Piccioni E, Manicone PF, Berardi D, Perfetti G, Calviello G. N-3 polyunsaturated fatty acid effect in periodontal disease: state of art and possible mechanisms involved. *Int. J. Immunopathol. Pharmacol.* 2008;21(2):261-6.

Ramesh A, Mahajan K, Thomas B, Shenoy N, Bhandary R. Alveolar bone mass in pre- and postmenopausal women with serum calcium as a marker: a comparative study. *Indian J. Dent. Res.* 2011;22(6):878.

Rao PK, Reddy RV, Mapare SA, Nag VR, Gowtham K, Arora D. An investigation of blood hemogram and estimation of serum iron and protein levels in aggressive periodontitis patients: a clinic biochemical study. *J. Contemp. Dent. Pract.* 2013;14(5):852-7.

Reynolds MA, Dawson DR, Novak KF, Ebersole JL, Gunsolley JC, Branch-Mays GL, Holt SC, Mattison JA, Ingram DK, Novak MJ. Effects of caloric restriction on inflammatory periodontal disease. *Nutrition.* 2009;25(1):88-97.

Riant E, Waget A, Cogo H, Arnal JF, Burcelin R, Gourdy P. Estrogens protect against high-fat diet-induced insulin resistance and glucose intolerance in mice. *Endocrinology.* 2009;150(5):2109-17.

Ritchie CS, Joshipura K, Hung HC, Douglass CW. Nutrition as a mediator in the relation between oral and systemic disease: associations between specific measures of adult oral health and nutrition outcomes. *Crit. Rev. Oral Biol.* M 2002;13(3):291-300.

Rodrigues VP, Libério SA, Lopes FF, Thomaz EB, Guerra RN, Gomes-Filho IS, Pereira AL. Periodontal status and serum biomarkers levels in haemodialysis patients. *J. Clin. Periodontol.* 2014;41(9):862-8.

Rosenstein ED, Kushner LJ, Kramer N, Kazandjian G. Pilot study of dietary fatty acid supplementation in the treatment of adult periodontitis. *Prostaglandins Leukot Essent Fatty Acids.* 2003;68(3):213-8.

Samnieng P, Ueno M, Shinada K, Zaitsu T, Wright FA, Kawaguchi Y. Oral health status and chewing ability is related to mini-nutritional assessment results in an older adult population in Thailand. *J. Nutr. Gerontol. Geriatr.* 2011;30(3):291-304.

Sanders AE, Slade GD, Fitzsimmons TR, Bartold PM. Physical activity, inflammatory biomarkers in gingival crevicular fluid and periodontitis. *J. Clin. Periodontol.* 2009;36(5):388-95.

Schenker S. Undernutrition in the UK. British Nutrition Foundation Bulletin 2003;28 :87-120.

Scientific Report of the 2015 Dietary Guidelines Advisory Committee. Retrieved on March 18, 2015 at http://health.gov/dietaryguidelines/2015-scientific-report/PDFs/Scientific-Report-of-the-2015-Dietary-Guidelines-Advisory-Committee.pdf

Sculley DV, Langley-Evans SC. Salivary antioxidants and periodontal disease status. *P. Nutr. Soc.* 2002;61(1):137-43.

Senoo K, Lane D, Lip GY. Stroke and bleeding risk in atrial fibrillation. *Korean Circ J.* 2014;44(5):281-90.

Shimazaki Y, Shirota T, Uchida K, Yonemoto K, Kiyohara Y, Iida M, Saito T, Yamashita Y. Intake of dairy products and periodontal disease: the Hisayama Study. *J. Periodontol.* 2008;79(1):131-7.

Shinkawa T, Hayashida N, Mori K, Washio K, Hashiguchi K, Taira Y, Morishita M, Takamura N. Poor chewing ability is associated with lower mucosal moisture in elderly individuals. Tohoku *J. Exp. Med.* 2009;219(4):263-7.

Shukla A, Kumar K, Singh A. Association between obesity and selected morbidities: a study of BRICS countries. *PLoS One.* 2014 Apr 9;9(4):e94433.

Sidi A, Ashley F. Influence of frequent sugar intakes on experimental gingivitis. *J. Periodontol.* 1984; 55: 419-423.

Singh N, Chander Narula S, Kumar Sharma R, Tewari S, Kumar Sehgal P. Vitamin E supplementation, superoxide dismutase status, and outcome of scaling and root planing in patients with chronic periodontitis: a randomized clinical trial. *J. Periodontol.* 2014;85(2):242-9.

Singh R. Food and Nutrition for Nurses. 2012, Jaypee Brothers Medical Publishers.

Slade EW Jr., Bartuska D, Rose LF, Cohen DW. Vitamin E and periodontal disease. *J. Periodontol.* 1976;47(6):352-54.

Staudte H, Güntsch A, Völpel A, Sigusch BW. Vitamin C attenuates the cytotoxic effects of Porphyromonas gingivalis on human gingival fibroblasts. *Arch. Oral Biol.* 2010;55(1):40-5.

Staudte H, Kranz S, Völpel A, Schütze J, Sigusch BW. Comparison of nutrient intake between patients with periodontitis and healthy subjects. *Quintessence Int.* 2012 Nov-Dec;43(10):907-16.

Staudte H, Sigusch BW, Glockmann E. Grapefruit consumption improves vitamin C status in periodontitis patients. *Br. Dent. J.* 2005 Aug 27;199(4):213-7, discussion 210.

Stevens GA, Singh GM, Lu Y, Danaei G, Lin JK, Finucane MM, Bahalim AN, McIntire RK, Gutierrez HR, Cowan M, Paciorek CJ, Farzadfar F, Riley L, Ezzati M; Global Burden of Metabolic Risk Factors of Chronic Diseases Collaborating Group (Body Mass Index). National, regional, and global trends in adult overweight and obesity prevalences. *Popul. Health Metr.* 2012;10(1):22.

Strippoli GF, Palmer SC, Ruospo M, Natale P, Saglimbene V, Craig JC, Pellegrini F, Petruzzi M, De Benedittis M, Ford P, Johnson DW, Celia E, Gelfman R, Leal MR, Torok M, Stroumza P, Bednarek-Skublewska A, Dulawa J, Frantzen L, Ferrari JN, del Castillo D, Hegbrant J, Wollheim C, Gargano L; ORAL-D Investigators. Oral disease in adults treated with hemodialysis: prevalence, predictors, and association with mortality and adverse cardiovascular events: the rationale and design of the ORAL Diseases in hemodialysis (ORAL-D) study, a prospective, multinational, longitudinal, observational, cohort study. *BMC Nephrol.* 2013;14:90.

Suresh S, Mahendra J. Multifactorial relationship of obesity and periodontal disease. *J. Clin. Diagn. Res.* 2014;8(4):ZE01-3.

Suvan J, D'Aiuto F, Moles DR, Petrie A, Donos N. Association between overweight/obesity and periodontitis in adults. A systematic review. *Obes. Rev.* 2011;12(5):e381-404.

Tanaka K, Miyake Y, Sasaki S, Ohya Y, Miyamoto S, Matsunaga I, Yoshida T, Hirota Y, Oda H; Osaka Maternal and Child Health Study Group. Magnesium intake is inversely associated with the prevalence of tooth loss in Japanese pregnant women: the Osaka Maternal and Child Health Study. *Magnes Res.* 2006;19(4):268-75.

Tanzer JM, Grant LP, McMahon T, Clinton D, Eanes ED. Simultaneous caries induction and calculus formation in rats. *J. Dent. Res.* 1993;72(5):858-64.

The Giessen Declaration. *Public Health Nutr.* 2005;8(6A):783-6.

Thomas B, Gautam A, Prasad BR, Kumari S. Evaluation of micronutrient (zinc, copper and iron) levels in periodontitis patients with and without diabetes mellitus type 2: a biochemical study. *Indian J. Dent. Res.* 2013;24(4):468-73.

Thomas B, Kumari S, Ramitha K, Ashwini Kumari MB. Comparative evaluation of micronutrient status in the serum of diabetes mellitus patients and healthy individuals with periodontitis. *J. Indian Soc.* Periodontol. 2010;14(1):46-9.

Thomas B, Ramesh A, Suresh S, Prasad BR. A comparative evaluation of antioxidant enzymes and selenium in the serum of periodontitis patients with diabetes mellitus type 2. *Contemp Clin. Dent.* 2013;4(2):176-80.

Tomofuji T, Ekuni D, Sanbe T, Irie K, Azuma T, Maruyama T, Tamaki N, Murakami J, Kokeguchi S, Yamamoto T. Effects of vitamin C intake on gingival oxidative stress in rat periodontitis. *Free Radic. Biol. Med.* 2009;46(2):163-8.

Traversy G, Chaput JP. Alcohol Consumption and Obesity: An Update. *Curr Obes. Rep.* 2015;4(1):122-130.

Tucker S. Food and Nutrition for Nurses. Prentice Hall; 1 edition, 2010, pg. 17-18.

Turnbaugh PJ, Bäckhed F, Fulton L, Gordon JI. Diet-induced obesity is linked to marked but reversible alterations in the mouse distal gut microbiome. *Cell Host Microbe.* 2008;3(4):213-23.

Turnbaugh PJ, Ridaura VK, Faith JJ, Rey FE, Knight R, Gordon JI. The effect of diet on the human gut microbiome: a metagenomic analysis in humanized gnotobiotic mice. *Sci Transl Med.* 2009;1(6):6ra14.

Van der Velden U, Kuzmanova D, Chapple IL. Micronutritional approaches to periodontal therapy. *J. Clin. Periodontol* 2011;38 Suppl 11:142-58.

Walls AW, Steele JG. The relationship between oral health and nutrition in older people. *Mech. Ageing Dev.* 2004;125(12):853-7.

Wang L, Wang J, Jin Y, Gao H, Lin X. Oral administration of all-trans retinoic acid suppresses experimental periodontitis by modulating the Th17/Treg imbalance. *J. Periodontol.* 2014;85(5):740-50.

Watanabe K, Cho YD. Periodontal disease and metabolic syndrome: a qualitative critical review of their association. *Arch. Oral Biol.* 2014;59(8):855-70.

Weinberg MA, Bral M. Laboratory animal models in periodontology. *J. Clin. Periodontol.* 1999;26(6):335-40.

Wirt A, Collins CE. Diet quality--what is it and does it matter? *Public Health Nutr.* 2009;12(12):2473-92.

World Health Organisation European Region. Food based dietary guidelines in the WHO European Region. Copenhagen: WHO, Europe, 2003 - www.euro.who.int/Document /E79832.pdf

World Health Organization. Diet, Nutrition, and the Prevention of Chronic Diseases. Report of a WHO/FAO Consultation. Geneva: WHO Technical Report Series 916; 2002

Wu W, Yang N, Feng X, Sun T, Shen P, Sun W. Effect of vitamin C administration on hydrogen peroxide-induced cytotoxicity in periodontal ligament cells. *Mol. Med. Rep.* 2015;11(1):242-8.

Wyss C, Guggenheim B. Effects of the association of conventional rats with Actinomyces viscosus Nyl and Bacteroides gingivalis W83. *J. Periodontal. Res*. 1984;19(6):574-7.

Yamazaki Y. Effects of destructive periodontitis, induced by diet, on the mechanical properties of the periodontal ligament of the mandibular first molar in golden hamsters. *J. Periodontal. Res.* 1992;27(2):149-58.

Yamori M, Njelekela M, Mtabaji J, Yamori Y, Bessho K. Hypertension, periodontal disease, and potassium intake in nonsmoking, nondrinker african women on no medication. *Int. J. Hypertens.* 2011;2011:695719.

Yan Y, Zeng W, Song S, Zhang F, He W, Liang W, Niu Z. Vitamin C induces periodontal ligament progenitor cell differentiation via activation of ERK pathway mediated by PELP1. *Protein Cell.* 2013;4(8):620-7.

Yoshihara A, Iwasaki M, Miyazaki H. Mineral content of calcium and magnesium in the serum and longitudinal periodontal progression in Japanese elderly smokers. *J. Clin. Periodontol.* 2011;38(11):992-7.

Zare Javid A, Seal CJ, Heasman P, Moynihan PJ. Impact of a customised dietary intervention on antioxidant status, dietary intakes and periodontal indices in patients with adult periodontitis. *J. Hum. Nutr. Diet.* 2014;27(6):523-32.

Zhan Y, Samietz S, Holtfreter B, Hannemann A, Meisel P, Nauck M, Völzke H, Wallaschofski H, Dietrich T, Kocher T. Prospective Study of Serum 25-hydroxy Vitamin D and Tooth Loss. *J. Dent. Res.* 2014;93(7):639-644.

Zhang X, Meng H, Sun X, Xu L, Zhang L, Shi D, Feng X, Lu R, Chen Z. Elevation of vitamin D-binding protein levels in the plasma of patients with generalized aggressive periodontitis. *J. Periodontal. Res.* 2013;48(1):74-9.

Zhang X, Meng H, Xu L, Zhang L, Shi D, Feng X, Lu R, Chen Z. Vitamin d-binding protein levels in plasma and gingival crevicular fluid of patients with generalized aggressive periodontitis. *Int. J. Endocrinol.* 2014;2014:783575.

Zhou X, Han J, Song Y, Zhang J, Wang Z. Serum levels of 25-hydroxyvitamin D, oral health and chronic obstructive pulmonary disease. *J. Clin. Periodontol.* 2012;39(4):350-6.

In: Oral Health
Editor: Julia Renee Barnes
ISBN: 978-1-63482-832-1

Chapter IV

Oral Health Literacy As a Social Determinant of Oral Health

R. Constance Wiener, MA, DMD, PhD
West Virginia University, School of Dentistry,
Department of Dental Practice and Rural Health;
School of Public Health, Department of Epidemiology,
Morgantown, WV

Abstract

Biological, psychological, sociological, and ecological features of life contribute and interact simultaneously in the development of an individual's oral health. For example, a person's oral health is influenced by culture/race/ethnicity, neighborhood/rural area, government structure (with programs for education and healthcare), and level of social cohesion/power (support from friends, family, church members, community members, etc.), all of which may vary over the person's life, *as well as* brushing and flossing, proper nutrition, immunological status, saliva production, oral microbes, etc. When group variations in preventable disease differ primarily due to social conditions, the situation is described as a health disparity due to the social determinants of health.

In the U.S., public policymakers are expected to address such group health differences through: the promotion of education; safe/healthy homes, schools, and workplaces; reduction of poverty; and the reduction of discrimination (racial-based, gender-based, age-based, etc.) in addition to: the encouragement of life-style changes to lessen risk; healthcare; and research.

The purpose of this chapter is to review the influence of improved oral health literacy considering the circumstances in which a person has been born, lives, and works (social determinants), the microbiological mechanisms, and the public's influence to improve oral health.

Introduction

Definitions

The World Health Organization (WHO, 2008) defined *social determinants of health* as the "circumstances in which people are born, grow up, live, work, and age, as well as the systems put in place to deal with illness. These circumstances are in turn shaped by a wider set of forces: economics, social policies, and politics."

The National Institute of Dental and Craniofacial Research (NIDCR, 2005)defined *oral health literacy* as the "degree to which individuals have the capacity to obtain, process and understand basic oral health information and services needed to make appropriate health decisions." The Calgary Charter on Literacy (2011) further included in the definition, a professional's role in listening, explaining and verifying that the person receiving the message understands the health message provided. A person may be educated, but have limited oral health literacy; or have a limited education and have high oral health literacy. Education and oral health literacy are not sufficient in and of themselves for good oral health.

Epidemiology

The U.S. is a culture with high literacy and skill demands (Nielsen-Bohlman, et al., 2004). People are asked to perform disease management skills for themselves and the people in their care which may involve activities that would have been performed by skilled professionals in the recent past including blood pressure monitoring, wound management, home chemotherapy regimens, and home discharge care for out-patient surgeries among others. There are 90 million Americans with limited literacy skills (Nielsen-Bohlman, et al., 2004) in a population of 319 million (U.S. Census, 2014). In the National Assessment of Adult Health Literacy, 2003, 19,000 adults, ages 16 years and above, were tested for health literacy. Fourteen percent had below basic health literacy; 22% had basic health literacy; 53% had intermediate health literacy, and 12% had proficient health literacy (Kutner, et al., 2006). The financial burden associated with limited health literacy is $106 billion to $238 billion annually, or between 7-17% percent of healthcare expenditures (Vernon et al., 2007). Limited health literacy has somatic consequences. It has been associated with:

- poorer health outcomes (Oramasionwu, et al., 2014);
- less use of preventive care (Chen, et al., 2013);
- more emergent care needs (Griffey, et al., 2014);
- errors in medication usage (O'Conor, et al., 2014); and
- misunderstandings in providing consent for treatment and/or research.

Seeking and obtaining dental care are important in oral health. Many people who do not have adequate health literacy do not ask for help in obtaining information, or have not developed a vocabulary to navigate the healthcare system (Schwartzberg, et al., 2005). The role of oral health literacy in seeking and obtaining dental care is explored in this chapter.

Theoretical Framework

Theoretical frameworks are used to explain what people observe as well as what is not considered. In one current theory about health, the ecosocial theory, Krieger (2011) proposed that the theoretical framework to explain health must not be reduced simply to biological mechanisms (a reductionist model), since rates and patterns are known to change and the changes cannot be adequately explained simply by a biopsychosocial model (Yamada & Palmer, 2007); and health cannot be fully explained by how society/employers/ governments/insurance companies, etc., interact with people. Instead, she theorized an Ecosocial Theory of Health which is dependent upon:

- "The cumulative interplay of exposure, susceptibility, and resistance across the lifecourse;"
- embodiment (the internalization) of the influences around oneself;
- pathways of how various exposures (such as trauma, hunger, stress, toxins, tobacco, bullying, access to healthcare, etc.) become internalized; and
- accountability and agency (how society addresses disparities) (Karger, 2011). The Krieger Ecosocial Theory of Health is the theoretical framework for this chapter.

Historical Perspective

During the 1950's, with the introduction of fluoride toothpastes, there was an advancement in dental caries control through the biological mechanism by which fluoride acts, as well as an effort to influence the large cohort of children born after World War II to brush and floss and thereby use the fluoride toothpastes. There was an internalization of the need to brush and floss by the dental professional community as well as the public at large. There were many stakeholders. Dental hygienists and dentists discussed prevention with patients, and teachers and school nurses in elementary schools taught lessons on tooth anatomy, caries (cavities), and nutrition. Teachers asked students to record the number of times they brushed/flossed during a week as homework assignments. Many school board members budgeted toothbrushes, toothpaste, and disclosing tablets for students. Many state legislators mandated oral evaluations and surveillance of children in specific grades after which the results were aggregated and forwarded to state health departments. Fluoride toothpaste was heavily marketed on television. Many community leaders mandated fluoride to be added to drinking water. Important positive changes occurred that improved oral health. Advancement in oral health (through community water fluoridation) was considered one of the top 10 public health improvements in the 20th century (CDC, 2013). There was a social movement with many people involved to improve oral health; people were motivated to receive and act upon the message.

Through the years, there were changes. Some school board members in various communities agreed to add fluoride rinse programs, school dental programs, and topical fluoride programs. Other school board members in other communities discontinued the programs, and discontinued providing disclosing tablets as some parents and teachers complained that they were inconvenient, messy, and stained clothes. Some states legislators did not recognize the value of surveillance. As a result, some surveillance programs were discontinued. The emphasis on oral health education and prevention waned in schools as pressure to spend time on other aspects of education increased.

There were fewer voices reinforcing the importance of oral health. Dentists and dental hygienists continued to speak to groups as well as with patients individually about the need for preventive care. Although the message was to a smaller number of people, members of dental organizations continued to work toward policies to improve oral health and researchers made many advances in improving restorative materials and dental sealants. There have been fluctuations in dental visits for professional care, but the overall trend has been positive. In a nationally representative study conducted in 1965, 46% of the participants self-reported having had a dental visit within the year (O'Shea & Gray, 1968). In 2012, the number was 67.2% in a similar national study (of the states and Washington, DC), the Behavioral Risk Factor Surveillance System survey (BRFSS, 2013). The U.S. Department of Health and Human Services used a different data source, the Medical Expenditure Panel (MEP), to develop health goals for 2020. For oral health, one of the Healthy Person 2020 objectives was to improve the number of dental visits within the year from 44.5%, the 2007 MEP baseline, to 49.0% (HealthyPeople.gov, 2014).

Whether the percentage of people in the U.S. who have *not* had a dental visit within the year is more than 30%, or more than 50%, neither situation should be acceptable. Dentists conducting biannual dental examinations have found incipient caries, incipient periodontitis (bone, ligament and gum tissue loss around teeth) and have intervened to improve patient health. Moreover, dentists conducting head and neck cancer screenings have identified early signs of oral and head and neck cancers. These cancers account for 6% of all malignancies in the United States (American Academy of Otolaryngology, 2014). Early intervention is important. Therein lies the role of oral health literacy as a social determinant of oral health, that is, oral health literacy is "needed to make appropriate health decisions," among which is dental care (NIDCR, 2005).

Embodiment; Pathways to Embodiment; Interplay of Exposure/ Susceptibility/Resistance

Each individual incorporates his or her culture/society into himself/herself. (A person is simultaneously his/her race, ethnicity, class, gender, and sex) (Krieger, 2011). Until recently, it was difficult to consider such subgroups of the population in research. The statistical tests to delve into subgroup differences became possible with computers with fast processing capabilities and large databases. Asking the right questions, selecting the right variables, and using the right statistical analyses are important concerns in research as data can be parsed and associations found which may be spurious, happenstance, biased, confounded, and/or wrong if the examination is flawed.

Studying populations has many vagarities. People and societies change. Their practices and habits change. For example, in terms of concerns which influence dental care, the types of food and the nature of food consumption in the U.S. has been changing. Fast food meals and meals prepared away from home have been rapidly increasing from 25.9% in 1970 to 43.1% in 2012, due in part to the number of women employed outside the home, higher family incomes, affordability, convenience (Lin, 2014), long commute times, after school activities, etc. Food away from home is often calorie dense and nutritionally deficient (Lin, 2014). The food tends to be higher in fat, and lower in calcium, fiber, and iron (Lin, 2014; Berge, et al., 2014) and higher in sugar. Commercially pre-packaged foods, pre-packaged ready-to-use items (pie crusts, cookie dough, etc.), recipes simplified to use pre-packaged/modified ingredients, and foods prepared away from home have become culturally "traditional" for many people.

Sugary drinks have also increased over the last 30 years. Half of the population over age two drinks a sugary drink on any given day (O'Conor, et al., 2014). (Males drink an average of 178 calories from sugary drinks daily; females drink an average of 103 calories from sugary drinks daily) (O'Conor, et al., 2014). Non-Hispanic black children have 8.5% of their calories from sugary drinks; Mexican Americans have 7.4% of their calories from sugary drinks (O'Conor, et al., 2014). Children living in homes 0-130% of the Federal Poverty level have 8.2% of their calories from sugary drinks; children living at 350% of the Federal Poverty level have 6.7% of their calories from sugary drinks (O'Conor, et al., 2014).

The combination of refined foods and sugary drinks provides a sugary food source for the natural bacteria in the mouth (the oral microbiome), which produce acid. Saliva has an ability to reduce the effect of the acid, however the buffering capacity of saliva can be overwhelmed. If the saliva's buffers are overwhelmed, the acid can remove the calcium from teeth (demineralize the teeth). Additionally, an inflammatory response occurs within the tooth during the attack and once the bacteria penetrate the enamel and enter the softer dentin, they can establish a localized infection of the tooth (caries).

Greater physiological and psychological stress associated with work, school, home, trauma, discrimination, multimorbidities, and other conditions such as pregnancy and depression, have also been associated with increased inflammation. When bacterial plaque is not removed, bacteria may attack the tissue between the tooth and its supporting tissue, and an inflammatory response may occur in the tissue around the tooth and the tooth's supporting bone. The inflammatory response is often greater with the aforementioned conditions of physiological and psychological stress.

Additionally, patterns of eating and drinking frequently throughout the day, binge eating, eating when not hungry, eating away from family/friends, and eating in front of the television may also influence oral hygiene habits. Being away from home, tired, disbelieving in the need for oral hygiene, having no oral hygiene aids, or being unaware of the need to brush and floss decreases the probability of removing plaque and increases the possibilities of dental caries and periodontitis.

Accountability and Agency Related to Poor Oral Health

Since there are many contributing factors associated with poor oral health, there are also many approaches that may improve oral health. Krieger, in her ecosocial theory, suggests that *only* focusing on lifestyle or individual factors (such as telling people to brush, floss, avoid frequent consumption of sugary drinks, etc. where oral health is concerned) limits the research to biomedical individualism and removes the context in which a person lives from the analysis (decontextualizes the analysis) (Krieger, 2008). Similarly *only* focusing on society and change in production and distribution to improve health, (such as removing soda machines from schools; including high fructose corn syrup listings on packaging, placing calorie lists on restaurant menus/menu boards, etc.) limits the research to social hierarchies (Krieger, 2008). Both are needed.

In addressing accountability, one question to consider is who benefits, (qui bono) from people having poor oral health or the conditions which lead to poor oral health and who will be hurt by a change in the status quo? Although dental professionals treat the results of poor oral health and benefit financially from such care, many take an ethical oath to do no harm and to not over-treat. Manufacturers of professional dental products, dental devices, and specialized dental equipment benefit with the status quo. Producers and sellers (from grocery store owners, convenience store owners, to restaurateurs) of high sugar or high fructose corn syrup laden products could be hurt financially by a change in purchasing patterns if people would eat fewer refined carbohydrates. Strategies such as labeling high fructose corn syrup differently (such as DAHLIA syrup, isoglucose, glucose-fructuose, crystalline fructose, tapioca syrup, corn glucose fructose syrup, or corn sugar) are being used for obfuscation.

However, U.S. dental insurance companies, the U.S. government paying for dental care in programs such as Medicaid, employers paying for dental insurance, the military (needing military preparedness), and producers of toothpastes, tooth brushes, floss, mouth rinses, and other oral health-related products would benefit from improved oral health. Dental professionals would have a change in services, but many want the people in their care to have improved oral health; additionally improved communication and dental literacy lessens the exposure to malpractice claims as people understand the procedures and potential consequences (Riess & Kraft-Todd, 2014).

It should be noted that although effective communication is necessary for good healthcare, professional students with negative attitudes toward learning communication skills undervalue or devalue the skills in their clinical practice and are less knowledgeable concerning patient-professional interactions than students with positive attitudes (Wright, et al., 2006). In an unpublished pilot study of dental students, those who valued communication skills in practice learned more from a didactic course in communication (McKenzie, 2014). In a follow-up study of dental students, a single didactic course in communication had no significant effect on student attitudes or self-assessment (McKenzie, 2014). In a study of medical students, female medical students had more positive attitudes toward communication skills education than male medical students, while male students had higher scores in their perceived competence and confidence about communicating than female students (Wright, et al., 2006). Medical students having had clinical experience, reported higher positive attitudes toward communication skills training than students who had yet to have clinical experience (Wright, et al., 2006). These attitudes are barriers to quality healthcare.

There are also barriers in dental literacy resulting from stereotypes and perceptions of dentists held by many people. In most movies, dentists are portrayed as mean, scary, sadistic, immoral, unethical, and corrupt individuals (Glazman, 2014). The public blames dentists for the inadequacies in policies, for being greedy, and uncompassionate (Glazman, 2014). Dentists are under the pressure of having rising equipment costs, educational costs, and dental spending below the rate of inflation (Carter, 2014) while assigned fees are not keeping pace with the amount of work that is being done (Skalsky LJ, 2014; Glazman, 2014). As many dentists turn the focus of their practice to cosmetic bleaching, Botox, couture veneers, etc., dentistry is demedicalized (Glazman, 2014). Dental professionals need to manage their practices as businesses, while providing quality care and having communication skills to explain treatment needs in an honest and ethical manner. However, if the public distrusts dentists, the communication and oral health literacy needed will fall short of the action required for quality healthcare.

Nevertheless, many groups encourage agency/action toward quality oral healthcare. Successful, quality healthcare involves cognitive knowledge, technical skills, and the ability to create rapport and a therapeutic relationship through social skills (among other variables) (Orsini & Jerez, 2014). Improving another person's health literacy is one aspect of social skills.

Where oral health literacy is considered, there are opportunities for many people to become involved in increasing oral health literacy and improving oral health as well as working to improve individual efforts toward good oral health within the social context. School board members, teachers, public health officials, dentists, hygienists and others can impact the knowledge, attitudes, and beliefs of students and the public at large to whom they are responsible through education and familiarizing people with medical terminology as well as using words that are easier to understand. One U.S. government initiative toward improving understanding is the 2010 Plain Writing Act in which the government must have "clear communication that the public can use and understand" in its documents (Plain Language, http://www.plainlanguage.gov/plLaw/index.cfm). Policy makers at the U.S. National Institutes of Health (NIH) also support the use of plain language. Plain language is described at the NIH website as being grammatically correct and professional (NIH, 2013). Plain language is also described at the website as *not* being "dumbed down" (NIH, 2013). Plain language is clear communication which helps people to understand (NIH, 2013). Health literacy is a part of the plain language initiative of the NIH. At the National Oral Health Conference in 2010, the American Dental Association (ADA) developed a set of goals and a plan for improved oral health literacy for 2010-2015 (Podschun, 2012). Throughout the nation, efforts are underway in educating professionals about communication techniques to improve oral health literacy.

Research in Health Literacy/Health Literacy Communications

Objective Measures: Screenings and Grade level evaluations

Health literacy may be considered a construct which cannot be measured directly (a latent variable). Many researchers have suggested a variety of techniques to measure health literacy (Parker, et al., 1995; Baker, et al., 1999; Kutner, et al., 2008; Davis, et al., 1993). Many involve reading word lists.

However, there are many concerns about conducting health literacy screenings to determine who has a high literacy level and who has a low literacy level. Poor health literacy is associated with shame and embarrassment (Parikh, et al., 1996) and asking people to complete a health literacy test may increase the shame and embarrassment to the point of avoiding needed care. Many people hide their limited oral health literacy and would not be willing to participate in such activities or research. The tests have the confounders of medications, vision, stress, crying, accents, and distractions, among others; therefore the usefulness of testing is brought into question (Schwartzberg, et al., 2005). There are also concerns as to how and where the test results would be kept, and how the test would change treatment or care, if at all (Schwartzberg, et al., 2005). Recommendations exist in which the tests should not be used in a clinical setting unless tailored communication plans are intended (Davis, et al., 1998).

It is known that certain groups are considered more vulnerable to limited oral health literacy, such as individuals who have: English as a second language; chronic illness/disability; financial challenges; challenges with age, challenges with being pregnant, challenges with place of residence; challenges with having been incarcerated, etc. (Rivara, et al., 2011). Also the health literacy of typically high health literate individuals may be affected by pain, medication, illness, and finances (Evans, 2013).

As a result, there has been a shift: *all* people are considered to need plain language in communications; in instructions in medications; in lay brochures, pamphlets, and at official websites of medical and dental organizations and health related government websites. *Organizations and healthcare personnel* are charged with being health literate.

In terms of objective measures and evaluation, written communications, health communication brochures and pamphlets, and written items available on the internet should be possible to assess. Such documents are considered inappropriate when jargon or uncommon terminology is presented without also having explanations in the text, when too many poly-syllabic words are present, small font, or san serif typeset is used in the document, and when the communication is outdated or of poor quality (Wiener & Wiener-Pla, 2011). Accuracy of message is particularly important (Wiener & Wiener-Pla, 2013).

There are several measures which may be used to evaluate the reading level of brochures and pamphlets. Some of the methods can be done with software features that test the document's readability, however other methods require manual word and sentence counts. The most common tests are the are the Flesch Reading Ease test, the Flesch-Kincaid Grade level test, and the McLaughlin SMOG Readability Formula.

The Flesch Reading Ease test score is an analysis in which researchers determine the average sentence length, and the average number of syllables per word to score a document (Office Online, 2007). Scores between 60 and 70 indicate that the document is a standard document, and higher scores reflect greater reading ease (Office Online, 2007). The formula is:

Readability score = 206.835 – (1.015 * Average sentence length) –
(84.6 * Average number of syllables per word) (Office Online, 2007).

The Flesch-Kincaid Grade level test is a test for the school grade associated with the reading level of the document. The formula is

Grade level score = -15.59 + (0.39 * Average sentence length) +
(11.8 * Average number of syllables per word) (Office Online, 2007).

The McLaughlin SMOG Readability Formula is more complex and involves a conversion table for the school grade associated with the reading level of the document. Thirty sentences are used to calculate the readability level. Ten sentences are drawn from the beginning, middle and end of the document. The number of words with 3 or more syllables is counted in the 30 sentences. The square root of the count (to the nearest 10) plus 3 is calculated and the corresponding number is located on the conversion table with the reading grade level. (Readability Formulas, nd).

A problem encountered with each of the tests is, after a polysyllabic term has been identified and explained, the term continues to be counted as a difficult term in the readability test. For example, the term, chronic obstructive pulmonary disease, may be presented with the acronym "COPD," or with the words, "lung disease" following it parenthetically as: chronic obstructive pulmonary disease (COPD, or lung disease). Similarly, the word, hypertension may be presented with the words "high blood pressure" following it parenthetically as: hypertension (high blood pressure). It is important that people can recognize scientific or medical terms after the terms have been introduced and explained in a brochure or pamphlet so that they can fully understand their conditions. In reading level analyses tests, the reading level will be higher if scientific or medical terms are used (even if they have been explained). This is an aspect of determining readability levels which needs to be addressed.

In addition to brochures, pamphlets, and websites, it is necessary that prescriptions, medication instructions, and medication package inserts are written clearly and in plain language. Many healthcare professionals now use software to write prescriptions to decrease the misinterpretation involved with a handwritten prescription. Also, many healthcare professionals avoid Latin terminology and Roman numerals, which were once de rigueur. This helps to avoid confusion. However, package inserts and secondary labels on prescription bottles are often written at high grade levels and in small font. Some medications look alike; some medications sound alike (Wong, 2014). Drug interactions are important considerations when people are on several medications. Medication labels may have wording which can be understood from several points of view.

Some people may have difficulty calculating when to take medications. For example, if the instructions are to take a medication "3 times a day," some people may not be able to calculate the hours in which the medication should be taken.

Some people do not understand what is meant by a "teaspoon." Some people do not understand why some medications can be discontinued when symptoms subside, and why others must be continued until all of the medication is used. Other areas of confusion are why some medications should be taken with food, and some should not be taken with food; why some medications should not be taken if the person cannot stand or sit upright for 30 minutes; or how much water to take with a medication. Medication compliance is identified by the World Health Organization as a significant world-wide problem (Sabate, 2003).

Many pharmacy school professors, and owners of pharmacies are increasingly having pharmacy students or pharmacists speak directly with people who have been given a prescription, particularly if it is a new prescription. They explain how and when to take the medication, and what additional effects may occur with the medication. They demonstrate the use of syringes, or devices such as inhalers. These actions are very important and constitute helping people to become health literate. Nevertheless, many of these activities are perfunctory or done too rapidly for individuals who need more time to assimilate what is being explained. This is particularly true in busy pharmacies.

Additionally, screening tools are being developed to use non-obtrusive data from medical/dental health histories to determine if an individual may be more vulnerable to having a medication problem (Claydon-Platt, et al., 2014). One such screening tool is to identify people with diabetes at increased risk for medication problems (Claydon-Platt, et al., 2014).

Much has been done, but much remains to be done as medication errors and non-compliance continue to be significant problems.

Subjective Measures: Standardized Patients, Professorial Evaluations, Surveys

Certain communication styles and techniques are established in rubrics for evaluating healthcare students in their interactions with standardized patients, or through professorial evaluations of healthcare students with their patients. Throughout the nation, simulation laboratories are being used to teach technical skills, as well as to help students learn to communicate with patients. Students are video-taped speaking with standardized patients. The standardized patient concept was introduced by Howard Barrows at the University of Southern California in 1963 (Beattie, et al., 2014). The standardized patients and the students' instructors have criteria upon which they grade the students. The students are debriefed as to how they could improve communications. With the simulations, the students have an opportunity to practice appropriate communication techniques while taking histories, providing instructions, and giving explanations to individuals who are older, younger, of a different race/ethnicity, of a different socioeconomic status, have hearing problems or cannot hear, need an interpreter, or speak only limited English, etc. One concern with evaluating dental and dental hygiene students is that most of the research in oral health literacy has used criteria in medicine and psychology, rather than specifically for dentistry (Orsini & Jerez, 2014). A dental practitioner-patient interaction skills tool has been developed recently which has 43 indicators to evaluate a dental student's communication skills (Orsini & Jerez, 2014). Its use may be very helpful in addressing needs specific to dentistry and dental hygiene.

One communication skill that students develop and for which they are evaluated in simulations is being at eye level with the person with whom they are speaking and maintaining eye contact during the communication. An environmental barrier which is frequently encountered in general office settings is the placement of a hard-wired computer which is needed to input health data by the healthcare person. In such cases, it is important for the healthcare provider to return his or her gaze and body position to the patient as often as possible despite the inconvenience. Dental and dental hygiene students should conduct patient instruction and have other discussions before the patient is reclined in the dental chair and return the patient to the seated position as much as possible during waits (waits for clinical instructor checks, waits for processing materials, etc.)

Oral healthcare personnel must speak clearly, slowly, and in plain English in their explanations to patients. People may be primarily visual learners, auditory learners, or kinesthetic learners. It is necessary to provide visual aids for visual learners, verbal explanations for auditory learners, and physical, touchable aids for kinesthetic learners. It is best to limit messages to two to three concepts at a time. The use of models is often helpful. Words or pictures drawn on notepads help patients to understand and remember complex information. Patients are helped when healthcare professionals verbally summarize brochures and pamphlets and highlight or underline important concepts as the professional is speaking with the patient. Over-the-counter medication recommendations should be provided in written form with proper dosing, either on the office's computer generated prescription form, or on a sheet from a prescription pad to emphasize the importance of the over-the-counter medication.

The students' clinical professors also determine if students are using behavior management techniques such as live/video modeling, tell-show-do, teach-back, positive reinforcement/encouragement, and motivational interviewing. Live modeling is a technique that is useful in working with children. Bandura (1967) defined modeling as a means to acquire behavior through the observation of a model (Farhat-McHayleh, et al., 2009). In a dental setting, a parent is asked to sit in the dental chair and undergo a short procedure, such as an examination, while the child observes and asks questions (Farhat-McHayleh, et al., 2009). Video modeling is similar, however the procedure is watched on a screen and the provider answers questions after the video is viewed.

Tell-show-do is another behavior management technique used in dentistry. Its antecedents are in World War I when Charles R. Allen developed the "preparation, presentation, application, test" model for preparing workers for specific jobs (Huntzinger, 2007; Allen, 1917). The presentation portion of his model was described as "tell, show, illustrate" and the application portion was described as "do" by the Bureau of Training, War Manpower Commission in 1944 (Huntzinger, 2007). Harold Addelston used the phrase "tell, show, do" to describe a direct interaction between the dental healthcare person and the patient in which the patient is told what will be done, is shown the instruments, or may receive a demonstration of how the instrument feels on the hand so that a sense of control is felt by the patient and the patient is not surprised by the procedure (Roberts, et al., 2010; Glazman, 2014; Hendrie, 2014).

Teach-back is a technique of checking that the message received was the one intended. The healthcare person says something to the effect of "I want to check that I have explained everything the way that I intended to explain it. Would you tell me how you are going to answer your family when they ask you about what I said to you?"(National Patient Safety Foundation, 2014).

In positive reinforcement/encouragement, the dental healthcare professional supports the patients' efforts to cooperate; he or she uses "I" statements and describes the situation. For example, an "I" statement to a child may have the form of: "I really like it when you keep your hands on your lap while I am working. It makes my job so much easier. Thank you." A descriptive statement may be: "Your hands have stayed in your lap for the whole procedure. What a good job at keeping your hands in your lap!"

Members of the National Patient Safety Foundation (2014) suggest providers need to teach patients to use "Ask me 3." Patients have the right to have these 3 important questions answered after a visit:

- What is my main problem?
- What do I need to do?
- Why is it important for me to do this?" (National Patient Safety Foundation, 2014).

Motivational interviewing is a technique to encourage changes to improve health (Miller & Rollnick, 2013). When people are considering change, they often need someone to discuss their situation and listen to their concerns. In the conversation, they need to address the reasons that they:

- want to change or modify a poor health behavior;
- the manner in which they will change to a healthier behavior; and,
- the importance of making the change to a healthier behavior.

A healthcare professional helps by listening. A healthcare professional helps by listening. Much of motivational interviewing is focusing the conversation on change, using open-ended questions, and listening. When the person has finished speaking, the healthcare professional summarizes the person's concerns and ambivalence, and then makes a reflective statement about what is being planned. The reflective statement would have the form of: "You plan to..;" or "You think you will..." followed by a rephrasing of what the person would like to accomplish. Motivational interviewing is often used with smoking cessation. Having their smoking patients consider smoking cessation or decrease the number of cigarettes smoked are concerns for dental professionals. Motivational interviewing has had mixed results in recent studies in smoking cessation and/or decreasing the number of cigarettes smoked (Mujika, et al., 2014; Ridner, et al., 2014; Pelletier, et al., 2014; Rohsenow, et al., 2014).

Other behavioral management techniques include voice modulation, distraction, asking for help in follow-up, nudges, and prompts. Certain words are commonly used when working with children to help alleviate their concerns about being in the dental office. Some examples are: "sleepy juice" instead of injection; "numbing jelly" instead of topical anesthetic; "Mr. Whistle" instead of high speed handpiece; and "Mr. Bumpy" instead of slow speed handpiece. It is important that the dental professional engages the parent/guardian to be supportive and that the parent or guardian avoids saying anxiety-provoking words, such as "shot" or "pulling teeth," or make comments that undermine the trust between the child and the healthcare professional.

To evaluate oral health literacy skills of dentists and dental hygienists after they have graduated is difficult. Outside of academia, the number of dental professionals who use the health literacy suggestions is only known through surveys of self-report. Self-reports are fraught with problems. The skills that are needed for health literacy competence are the same ones needed to evaluate competence, or any skill (Kruger & Dunning, 1999). People tend to overinflate self-appraisals (Kruger & Dunning, 1999); therefore, many researchers have eschewed using self-reports.

In one such self-report study, researchers determined that the most common communication technique used by participating Maryland dentists was the use of simple language (Maybury, et al., 2013). There were 93.4% of general dentists and 97.4% of pediatric dentists who reported using simple language (Maybury, et al., 2013). The second most common technique was to speak slowly; there were 77.4% of general dentists and 83.3% of pediatric dentists who reported speaking slowly (Maybury, et al., 2013).

A Walk through the Maze

Dentists and dental hygienists can improve their provision of oral health literacy within their clinical area by evaluating the steps needed to access their care. They should consider if their telephone is answered quickly. If telephone options are presented to the caller, they should decide if the options are clear or confusing. The office website should be evaluated for patient friendliness and easy navigability. Outdoor signs should be clear and have words that are easy to understand. The doctor's name should be listed on inside directories. Questions that should be considered are:

- Does the office staff member who presents forms to patients also offer to help?
- Are there policies in place for working with someone who does not speak English or who is deaf or hard of hearing?
- Do the brochures have plain language? Are they up to date? Is the font large enough for someone to read who has difficulty with vision?
- Are the models adequate to explain different oral conditions?
- Are there notepads to write explanations?
- Are oral dosing syringes prescribed or recommended for use rather than teaspoons?
- Are prescriptions written in such a way that there is little confusion about dosing?

Researchers recently studied 8,000 prescriptions and found that 73% had incomplete data (missing name, dosage form, dose and measuring unit, administration route, or intervals of administration); 15% had transcribing errors; 1/3 had administration errors; and there were 1.4-2.2% dispensing errors (Saghafi, & Zargarzadeh, 2014). Incomplete health histories, due to limited health literacy may also lead to errors in treatment. And difficulty navigating to the office may result in late or missed appointments.

Although a dental team may have good signage, easy to complete forms, and good brochures, there is also a need to walk through the maze of cultural differences. Many immigrants and non-native English speakers have cultural, religious, and dietary beliefs or views that may be different from the dental professional. It is important that the dental professional becomes familiar with the religious and cultural beliefs of the people they serve and develop cultural skills to improve communication. Different cultures have different metaphors and it is important to learn what patients mean when their descriptions use terminology and points of view from a different perspective.

Anticipatory Guidance: A Holistic Approach to Oral Health

The dental community is asked to provide anticipatory guidance through the life course. Even before pregnancy, women of childbearing age are encouraged by healthcare professionals to eat a healthful diet, to brush at least twice daily with fluoridated toothpaste, to floss daily, and to have routine dental care. Additionally, healthcare professionals are concerned about injury prevention, the need to wear seatbelts and to not engage in smoking, heavy drinking or illicit drug use. During pregnancy, expectant mothers are encouraged to have preventive care and to have needed emergency care in addition to proper nutrition and home care. Early in the pregnancy women may be advised to use toothpastes which are less bubbly to help with an increased gag reflex, and may be advised to limit snacking. Healthcare professionals encourage breastfeeding for the health and nutrition of babies for the first year of life. When solid food is introduced to infants, parents/guardians are advised to not blow on the baby's food, or share spoons or forks. If a pacifier is used, parents/guardians are advised not to place the pacifier in his or her mouth as bacteria from the parents may be transferred to the child if they do so. (Casamassimo & Holt, 2004). Pacifiers should be made as one unit of flexible, firm material; they should not be tied to the baby with a ribbon or string; and they should not be dipped into sugar/honey/syrup (Casamassimo & Holt, 2004). Anticipatory guidance in terms of injury prevention includes discussions with parents of newborns to place their baby to sleep on his or her back; to remove toys, bumper pads, etc. from the crib; to have a crib that meets current safety recommendations; to not put baby to bed with a bottle; to have the appropriate car seat; to avoid small items which may pose safety hazards (aspiration or swallowing); to keep one hand on the baby when he or she is on a high surface; and not to place the baby in a shopping cart (Casamassimo & Holt, 2004).

As the baby becomes a toddler, anticipatory guidance includes having the baby have his or her first dental visit by age one year. In the dental home, anticipatory guidance can be provided about nutrition, weaning, frequent snacking, limiting juices and sweet drinks as well as car seats and vaccinations. Parents/guardians should be asked to do a monthly screening of the child's teeth and be taught what would be considered suspicious. Parents/guardians need to know that children do not brush and floss adequately until age 6 or 7 and need help as well as supervision (ADA Division of Communications, 2002). A smear of toothpaste should be used until age 2; and a pea-sized amount of toothpaste should be used afterwards, at least twice daily. Injury prevention discussions may focus on having emergency contact information available; securing cabinets with household cleaners, medications, etc. inside, etc; keeping cords out of the reach of the child; using safety gates and toilet locks; keeping pet food/pet dishes away from the baby; and keeping the baby away from a pet while eating (Casamassimo & Holt, 2004). Parents should be advised that, should an injury to the face occur in which a primary tooth is lost, the primary tooth should not be re-implanted before the child is taken to the dentist. Anticipatory guidance also involves community activism to keep playgrounds and playground equipment maintained and safe (Casamassimo & Holt, 2004).

Through the years, discussions will need to continue about nutrition and daily oral health care. Older children begin to play sports, and sports injuries to the face and teeth are common. Therefore, a discussion of helmets and mouthguards is important. Parents spend a lot of money on sports shoes, but there is often reticence to spend the same amount of money on custom mouthguards. Custom mouthguards are as essential as specialty shoes. Should a permanent tooth be lost, parents/guardians should be prepared to gently rinse it with water, identify the front (facial) of the tooth and re-implant it before taking the child to the dentist. Adolescents often are under orthodontic care, and mouthguards are particularly necessary for teeth that are being moved. Also, for adolescents in orthodontic care, the need for good oral health care should be stressed by many people in the family and the child's dental health profession contacts.

Adolescents often engage in risk-taking behavior, therefore anticipatory guidance is needed in discussions with parents, and with adolescents concerning vehicular crashes, oral sequale which may be associated with oral sex, smoking, alcohol, and drug abuse and their effects on teeth and gingival tissue. Oral piercings and jewelry can fracture teeth, irritate and destroy gum (gingival) tissue. Dental healthcare professionals cannot assume that their adolescent patients are health literate from attending school, or having routine well child visits in which all of these topics have already been discussed. Although often difficult to breach this topic, bad breath also needs to be discussed. Many people find malodor socially offensive or disgusting and avoid people with bad breath. People may be unaware of the resulting social isolation. This is particularly important for adolescents.

As a person matures, the importance of oral health care often is considered in terms of aesthetics. Tooth whitening products are available as strips, gels, in toothpastes, sticks, and in dental offices. Their use and overuse should be discussed as anticipatory guidance.

Older adults who may be considering dentures need to have guidance in understanding the need for oral cancer screenings even after the dentures are in place, the need to evaluate the dentures for fit as there are bone changes over time, the potential for candida infections and angular cheilitis; the oral effects of common medications such as having a dry mouth, and altered taste, and nutritional needs.

Conclusion

Some people are fortunate. They have had daily oral hygiene practices from infancy; they have had routine care, and dental sealants; they have had any needed orthodontic care. Their circumstances and education have been bright and hopeful. Their smile and fresh breath may have helped them secure a job. Their genetics, nutrition, and oral microbiome are healthful.

Other people are not as fortunate. Drugs, alcohol, smoking, stress, trauma, discrimination, poor nutrition, bullying, social pressures, inadequate home care, as well as an acidogenic oral microbiome affected their oral health. The disparity involves social determinants in an ecosocial context.

Improving oral health literacy skills in oral healthcare professionals is one social policy among many which may help improve the nation's people's oral health and overall health.

References

ADA (American Dental Association) Division of Communications. Baby's first teeth. *JADA*. 2002;133:255.

Allen CR. The Instructor, the Man, and the Job. 1917. Lippencott, Philadelphia, PA. https://archive.org/details/instructormanjob00allerich.

American Academy of Otolaryngeology. 50 Facts about Oral, Head and Neck Cancer. 2014. http://www.entnet.org/?q=node/1501

Baker DW, Williams MW, Parker RM, Gazmararian JA, Nurss J. Development of a brief test to measure functional health literacy. *Patient Education and Counseling*. 1999;38:33-42.

Beattie BE, Kinney J, Fitzgerald M, Murdoch-Kinch CA, Guenther MK, Ridley K, Whitman L, Ramaswamy V. Dental and Dental Hygiene Students' Perceptions of a Standardized Patient Instructor Conflict Resolution Program. *JDE*. 2014;78:1397-1404.

Berge JM, Wall M, Hsueh TF, Fulkerson JA, Larson N, Neumark-Sztainer D. The Protective Role of Family Meals for Youth Obesity: 10-Year Longitudinal Associations. *J Pediatr*. 2014. DOI:10.1016/j.jpeds.2014.08.030.

BRFSS: Behavioral Risk Factor Surveillance System 2012 Codebook report. 2013. http://www.cdc.gov/brfss/annual_data/annual_2012.html

Carter SD. Dental Spending. *ADA News*. 2014;15:5.

Casamassimo P, Holt K., editors. Bright Futures in Practice: Oral Health Pocket Guide. Maternal and Child Health Bureau, U.S. Department of Health and Human Services. 2004. http://www.brightfutures.org/oralhealth/about.html

CDC (Centers for Disease Control and Prevention). Ten Great Public Health Achievements in the 20th Century. 2013. http://www.cdc.gov/about/history/tengpha.htm

Chen JZ, Hsu HC, Tung HJ, Pan LY. Effects of health literacy to self-efficacy and preventive care utilization among older adults. *Geriatr Gerontol Int*. 2013;13:70-76.

Claydon-Platt K, Manias E, Dunning T. Development and evaluation of a screening tool to identify people with diabetes at increased risk of medication problems relating to hypoglycaemia and medication non-adherence. *Contemporary Nurse.* 2014;48:10-25.

Coleman C, Kurtz-Rossi S, McKinney J, Pleasant A, Rootman I, Shohet L. The Calgary Charter on Health Literacy: Rationale and Core Principles for the Development of Health Literacy Curricula. 2011. Literacy, Information, and Communications System. http://www.centreforliteracy.qc.ca/sites/default/files/CFL_Calgary_Charter_2011.pdf

Davis TC, Long SW, Jackson RH, Mayeaux EJ, George RB, Murphy PW, Crouch MA. Rapid estimate of adult literacy in medicine: a shortened screening instrument. *Family Medicine*. 1993;25:391-395.

Davis TC, Michielutte R, Askow EN, Williams MV, Weiss BD. Practical assessment of adult literacy in healthcare. *Health Education and Behavior.* 1998;25:613-624.

Evans M. Providers help patients address emotion, money, health literacy. *Mod Healthcare.* 2013;43:16-18.

Farhat-McHayleh N, Harfouche A, Souaid P. Techniques for Managing Behaviour in Pediatric Dentistry: Comparative Study of Live Modelling and Tell–Show–Do Based on Children's Heart Rates during Treatment. *JCDA.* 2009;75:283-283f.

Glazman, J. Dental Anxiety: Personal and Media Influences on the Perception of Dentistry 2014. *Honors College Theses.* Paper 134. http://digitalcommons.pace.edu/honors college_theses/134

Griffey RT, Kennedy SK, McGownan L, Goodman M, Kaphingst KA. Is Low Health Literacy Associated with Increased Emergency Department Utilization and Recidivism? *Acad Emerg Med.* 2014;21:1109-1115.

HealthyPeople.gov Oral Health Objectives. U.S. Department of Health and Human Services, 2014. 200 Independence Avenue, S.W., Washington, DC 20201. http://www.healthy people.gov/2020/topics-objectives/topic/oral-health/objectives.

Hendrie F. Tell-Show-Do – It's not just for Children! Dental fear Central 2014. http://www.dentalfearcentral.org/help/psychology/tell-show-do/

Huntzinger J. The Roots of Lean Training Within Industry: The Origin of Japanese Management and Kaizen. 2007. Huntzinger summit presentation. http://twisummit.com /wp-content/uploads/2013/02/Roots-of-Lean-TWI1.pdf

Krieger N. *Epidemiology and the People's Health: Theory and Context.* 2011. Oxford press. New York, New York.

Krieger N. Proximal, Distal, and the Politics of Causation: What's Level Got to Do With It? *Am. J. Public Health.* 2008;98:221-230.

Kruger J, Dunning D. Unskilled and Unaware of It: How Difficulties in Recognizing One's Own Incompetence Lead to Inflated Self-Assessments. *Journal of Personality and Social Psychology.* 1999;77:1121-1134.

Kutner M,Greenberg E, Jin Y, Paulsen C. The health literacy of America's adults: results from the 2003 national assessment of adult literacy (NCES2006-483).Washington,DC: National Center for Education Statistics; 2006. http://nces.ed.gov/pubs2006/2006483.pdf.

Lin B. Food-Away-From-Home. U.S. Department of Agriculture. Food Consumption and Demand. http://www.ers.usda.gov/topics/food-choices-health/food-consumption-demand /food-away-from-home.aspx

McKenzie CT. Dental Student Attitudes Towards Communication Skills Instruction and Clinical Application. *JDE*. 2014;78:1388-1396.

Miller WR, Rollnick S. Motivational Interviewing helping people change. 2013 Guilford Press, New York, NY.

Mujika A, Forbes A, Canga N, de Irala J, Serrano I, Gasco P, Edwards M. Motivational interviewing as a smoking cessation strategy with nurses: an exploratory randomised controlled trial. *Int. J. Nurs Stud*. 2014;51:1074-82.

NIDCR (National Institute of Dental and Craniofacial Research), National Institutes of Health, US Public Health Service, US Dept of Health and Human Services. The invisible barrier: literacy and its relationship with oral health. A report of a workgroup sponsored by the National Institute of Dental and Craniofacial Research, National Institutes of Health, US Public Health Service, US Department of Health and Human Services. *J. Public Health Dent*. 2005;65:174–182.

NIH (National Institutes of Health). Plain language at NIH. 2013. http://www.nih.gov /clearcommunication/plainlanguage/index.htm

National Patient Safety Foundation. Ask me 3. 2014. http://www.npsf.org/?page=askme3

Nielsen-Bohlman L, Panzer AM, Kindig DA, Editors. Health Literacy: A Prescription to End Confusion. Committee on Health Literacy, Board on Neuroscience and Behavioral Health. Institute of Medicine of the National Academies. The National Academies Press. 2004. Washington, DC. http://www.nap.edu/openbook.php?record_id=10883&page=R1

O'Conor R, Wolf MS, Smith SG, Martynenko M, Vicencio DP, Sano M, Wisnivesky JP, Federman AD. Health Literacy, Cognitive Function, Proper Use and Adherence to Inhaled Asthma Controller Medications Among Older Adults with Asthma. *Chest*. 2014. doi: 10.1378/chest.14-0914.

Ogden CL, Kit BK, Carroll MD, Park S. Consumption of Sugar Drinks in the United States, 2005–2008. NCHS Data Brief. 2011;71 http://www.cdc.gov/nchs/data/databriefs/ db71.htm

Office online. Test your document's readability. https://support.office.com/en-us/article/Test-your-documents-readability-0adc0e9a-b3fb-4bde-85f4-c9e88926c6aa?ui=en-US&rs=en-US&ad=US

Oramasionwu CU, Bailey SC, Duffey KE, Shilliday BB, Brown LC, Denslow SA, Michalets EL. The Association of health literacy with time in therapeutic range for patients on warfarin therapy. *J. Health Commun*. 2014;19:19-28.

Orsini CA, Jerez OM. Establishing a Good Dentist-Patient Relationship: Skills Defined from the Dental Faculty Perspective. *JDE*. 2014;78:1405-1415.

O'Shea RM, Gray SB. Dental Patients' Attitudes and Behavior Concerning Prevention. *Public Health Reports* 1968;83:405-410.

Parker RM, Baker DW, Williams MV, Nurss JR. The Test of Functional Health Literacy in Adults: A New Instrument for Measuring Patients' Literacy Skills. *J. Gen. Intern Med*. 1995;10:537-541.

Parikh NS, Parker RM, Nurss JR, Baker DW, Williams MV. Shame and health literacy: the unspoken connection. *Patient Education and Counseling*. 1996;27:33-39.

Pelletier JH, Strout TD, Baumann. A systematic review of smoking cessation interventions in the emergency setting. *Am. J. Emerg Med*. 2014;32:713-724.

Plain Language: It's the law. http://www.plainlanguage.gov/plLaw/index.cfm

Podschun GD. National Plan to improve health literacy in dentistry. *J. Calif Dent Assoc.* 2012;40:317-20.

Readability Formulas. Grammatically writing support. http://www.readability formulas.com/smog-readability-formula.php

Ridner SL, Ostapchuk M, Cloud RN, Myers J, Jorayeva A, Ling J. Using motivational interviewing for smoking cessation in primary care. *South Med. J.* 2014;107:314-419.

Riess H, Kraft-Todd G. E.M.P.A.T.H.Y.: A Tool to Enhance Nonverbal Communication Between Clinicians and Their Clients. *Academic Medicine.* 2014;89:1108-1112.

Rivara FP, Erwin PC, Evans CA, Ganiats TG, Gehshan S, Geurink KV, et al., Committee on Oral Health Access to Services. Improving Access to Oral Health Care for Vulnerable and Underserved Populations. Institute of Medicine and National Research Council, 2011. Washington, DC: National Academies Press.

Board on Children, Youth, and Families, Board on Health Care Services, Institute on Medicine and National Research Council of the National Academies. 2011. The National Academies Press. Washington, DC. http://books.nap.edu/openbook.php?record_id =13116&page=R1

Roberts JF, Curzon MEJ, Koch G, Martens LC. Review: Behavior Management Techniques in Paediatric Dentistry. *European Archives of Paediatric Dentistry.* 2010;11:166-175.

Rohsenow DJ, Martin RA, Monti PM, Colby SM, Day AM, Abrams DB, Sirota AD, Swift RM. Motivational interviewing versus brief advice for cigarette smokers in residential alcohol treatment. *J. Subst Abuse Treat.* 2014;46:346-355.

Sabaté E., editor. Adherence to long term therapies: Evidence for action. WHO 2003. http://www.who.int/chp/knowledge/publications/adherence_report/en/

Saghafi F, Zargarzadeh AH. Medication error detection in two major teaching hospitals: What are the types of errors? *J. Res. Med. Sci.* 2014;19:617-23.

Skalsky IJ, PPO reimbursements. ADA News. 2014;5:5-6.

Wchwartzbert JG, Van Geest JB, Wang CC. Understanding Health Literacy. 2005. American Medical Association Press, U.S.

United States Census. U.S. and World Population Clock. 2014. http://www.census.gov/ popclock/

Vernon JA, Trujillo A, Rosenbaum S, DeBuono B. Low Health Literacy: Implications for National Health Policy. 2007. Washington, DC: Department of Health Policy, School of Public Health and Health Services, The George Washington University.

Wiener RC, Wiener-Pla. Evaluation of Educational Material for Tobacco Prevention and Cessation Used in West Virginia University Dental Programs. *The Journal of Dental Hygiene.*2011;85;204-210.

Wong ZS. Statistical classification of drug incidents due to look-alike sound-alike mix-ups. Health Informatics J. 2014. Nov 11. pii: 1460458214555040. (Epub ahead of print)

World Health Organization. Commission on Social Determinants of Health. Closing the gap in a generation: health equity through action on the social determinants of health. *Final Report of the Commission on Social Determinants of Health.* 2008. Geneva, World Health Organization.

Wright KB, Bylund C, Ware J, Parker P, Query JL, Baile W. Medical Student Attitudes Toward Communication Skills Training and Knowledge of Appropriate Provider-Patient Communication: A Comparison of First-Year and Fourth-Year Medical Students. *Med. Educ. Online.* 2006;11:18. http://www.med-ed-online.org.

Yamada S, Palmer W. An Ecosocial Approach to the Epidemic of Cholera in the Marshall Islands. *Social Medicine*. 2007;2:79-86.

In: Oral Health
Editor: Julia Renee Barnes
ISBN: 978-1-63482-832-1

Chapter V

Oral Health and Mental Health

Karen-Leigh Edward, PhD*
Director, St Vincent's Private Hospital Melbourne Nursing Research Unit
Associate Professor of Nursing Research, School of Nursing, Midwifery & Paramedicine| Australian Catholic University
Visiting Professor, School of Human & Health Sciences| University of Huddersfield, United Kingdom

Abstract

Mental disorders represent one of the largest burdens of disease globally. People who experience mental illness have incrementally worse physical health compared to the general population. While there is a movement in mental health care to consider physical health needs of service users, the oral health needs are not routinely assessed. Compounding the lack of routine or standardised oral health assessment in mental health services, service users/consumers often demonstrate avoidant health seeking behaviours. Health service avoidance for physical care needs is often compounded by prohibitive costs, stigma related to mental disorder, unsatisfactory previous encounters with oral care practitioners and psychiatric symptomatology impacting behaviours. This chapter will using contemporary literature describe the complexities related to oral care of people who experience mental disorders and the implications this may hold for their quality of life, practice, research and policy.

Keywords: Mental health, mental illness, oral effects of psychotropic medications, oral health, oral hygiene, periodontitis, xerostomia

* Mailing Address: Faculty of Health Sciences, Australian Catholic University, Melbourne Campus, Locked Bag 4115 FITZROY MDC 3065, Australia, T: +61 3 94117338, E: karen-leigh.edward@acu.edu.au

Introduction

This chapter will introduce you to the oral health needs of people experiencing mental illness. The chapter begins with an examination of co- occurring mental and physical health conditions with a focus on the oral condition of individuals. The assessment and intervention of oral health care will be discussed and a vignette will be offered to help the reader to assimilate their learning and reflect on their own practice. Some useful websites will be highlighted for the reader as points of reference to use for further learning.

Mental and Physical Health-Barriers to Care

Co-existing conditions are associated with poorer health outcomes and are characterised by higher rates of severe illness trajectory, frequent hospitalisations, higher rates of aggressive behaviour, relapse, suicidal behaviours, social isolation, family or care giver distress, homelessness and higher rates of mortality (Edward, Felstead, & Mahoney, 2012; Salamone, Yacoub, Mahoney, & Edward, 2013). While the physical health care of people who are receiving mental health services is a prominent focus of mental health care delivery, practice remains varied across countries and services. Some of the issues related to the lack of a standard approach to the physical care of people in mental health services relates to differences in governance, differences in funding support from governments for such initiatives and other impacts such as stigma and environmental barriers to receiving such care.

Oral Heath in People Who Live with Mental Illness

About 14% of the global burden of disease is attributed to mental illness (Prince et al., 2007; WHO, 2008). Among this number of people oral health care is not routinely sought by consumers or provided by mental health clinicians. Avoidant behaviours related to oral care and seeking an oral health practitioner presents as a significant barrier to help seeking behaviours of consumers. For example people who have had encounters with oral practitioners that were unsatisfactory or who found the costs associated with oral care prohibitive will postpone or avoid altogether attendance to receive oral care. Additionally, symptoms of mental illness such as amotivation, avolition, agitation or akathesia can also impact on the ability of the person to seek oral health consultation when in the community.

Up to 90% of people who have mental disorders receive medication management as part of their treatment. However, these drugs can impact the physical state of the individual and requires vigilant management by clinicians involved in the person's care. For example, the first generation antidepressant medications, tricyclic antidepressants (TCA's) were widely used and can bring about unwanted effects such as a dry mouth (xerostomia). This is related to the neurochemical actions of TCA's which block histaminic, cholinergic and alpha-1-adrenergic neuroreceptor sites. In the second generation antidepressants (such as serotonin reuptake inhibitors -SSRI's) the xerogenic impact is less than that seen in the TCA's. Dry mouth otherwise known as xerostomia occurs in 14% people taking SSRI's and 45% of people taking TCA's.

Mental disorders and the medications to treat these can be associated with common types of oral health concerns that the treating clinician can look for when undertaking a physical assessment of the individual. Common oral manifestations of major depression include: dental caries, poor oral hygiene, xerostomia, toothlessness, periodontal disease and poor nutrition (Edward, Hemingway, & Stephenson, 2012). The oral manifestations of the manic phase of bipolar affective disorder may include: worn down (abraded) oral mucosa and cervical tooth abrasion (due to over vigorous brushing or use of dental floss). In relation to antipsychotic medications the anticholinergic effects such as dry mouth experienced by up to 44% of patients.

People with mental disorders may choose unhealthy lifestyle choices or due to their own circumstance have fewer social supports or skills and as a result have higher rates of morbidity and mortality (Robson & Gray, 2007) and worse oral conditions (Persson, Axtelius, Söderfeldt, & Östman, 2009; Stevens, Spoors, Hale, & Bembridge, 2010). Such considerations commonly seen in people living with a mental illness can impact the person's oral condition for example taking psychoactive medications (Ponizovsky, Zusman, & Grinshpoon, 2009), smoking, poor diet, poor hydration and suboptimal hygiene behaviours. The prevalence of substance use disorders in people with early psychosis is relatively high with rates between 40-50% and the associated oral implications are substantial. The oral concerns related to substance abuse or misuse pertain to xerostomia (due to atrophy of the salivary glands), impaired wound healing due to liver damage, higher incidence of oral cancers due to heavy smoking and poor oral hygiene due to reduced brushing and flossing practices. Oral care is important to all people but especially those who experience mental disorders as poor oral condition can negatively impact the way in which the person relates to others in their social environment. Importantly, poor oral hygiene can amplify the prevalence of morbidity and mortality in patients (Berry, Davidson, Masters, & Rolls, 2007).

Oral bacteria, poor oral health care, and periodontitis appear to impact upon the incidence of infections (such as pneumonia), especially those infections acquired in a hospital (Paju & Scannapieco, 2007). The available evidence suggests systemic inflammation as seen in infections could represent a link between oral health and cardiovascular disease (CVD) (de Oliveira, Watt, & Hamer, 2010; Fisher, Borgnakke, & Taylor, 2010). A study of 11,000 adults highlights a significant increase in development of heart disease with people who only brushed their teeth once per day (de Oliveira, et al., 2010) as compared to those who brushed more. Importantly, cost efficient clinical care practices can alter patient outcomes, such as the implementation of a simple, low-cost oral care regime of flossing and brushing to decrease these risks for patients (Mori et al., 2006) where such interventions can also offer improvements in the persons quality of life (Buunk Werkhoven, Dijkstra, Schaub, Van Der Schans, & Spreen, 2010).

Oral Assessment in Mental Health Settings and Oral Condition Terminology

Oral assessment is not routinely undertaken in mental health in-patient or community settings. The reasons for this potentially relate to confusion related to roles of responsibility for oral care (clinician responsibility versus the consumer's responsibility), clinician and/or patient knowledge gaps related to oral conditions and confusing oral condition terminology (for example, the terms stomatitis and mucositis have been used interchangeably when describing inflammatory oral conditions). Finally there are a range of instruments available to undertake oral assessment however some require education in the first instance and generally few clinical staff outside of the speciality of oral health care are not provided undergraduate education related to the existence of such tools or the integration of such practices in routine care delivery.

Some of the available oral assessment instruments include the Oral Assessment Guide (OAG) (Eilers, Berger, & Petersen, 1987), the Oral Mucositis Index (OMI) (Eilers & Epstein, 2004), and the Oral Health Assessment Tool (OHAT) (Chalmers, King, Spencer, Wright, & Carter, 2005). Available oral health assessment tools often focus on the state of the mucosa including gingival, tongue, lips and the presence of breakdown or bleeding. The state of dentition is also often a focus where teeth are counted and surfaces are measured for signs of decay. Not all instruments take into consideration the social impacts of oral health problems or the ability of the consumer to self manage their oral care.

From the Mental Health Consumer's Perspective – Tony's Story

Tony has a diagnosis of schizophrenia and at 45 years old he has lived in the community independently for many years with the support of the local mental health community clinic. Tony lives alone and he has a case manager who visits him at home once a fortnight. Tony lives in a flat that is central to shops and public transport. He is on high dose antipsychotic medication to manage his psychotic condition and often experiences a dry mouth as an adverse effect of the medication. Tony has a brother who also has a mental illness and they don't see each other very often. His case worker notices Tony does not own a refrigerator and asks him how he keeps his food fresh. Tony says his diet consists of coffee, jam sandwiches and the occasional steak. Tony says he shops daily so there is no need for a fridge. He doesn't eat fruit or drink anything other than black coffee. Tony lives on a pension and smokes 2 packets of cigarettes per day.

Ask Yourself!

1. As the case worker do you think it is important to inspect Tony's oral condition during home visitations?
2. Who is the person to contact if Tony needs to have oral care needs addressed?
3. Is there any additional support you can offer Tony related to optimal oral care that he can perform himself?

Clinical reflection

Using the standard assessment forms available in mental health care provides an opportunity to assess and document the oral condition of mental health consumers.

The importance of inspecting oral condition in people who live with mental illness relates to – increasing the potential to retain teeth; early detection of poor oral health such as ulcers or even oral cancers; an opportunity to provide cost effective dental hygiene and potentially to identify where referral may be required.

Opening up dialogue with mental health consumers about their oral condition can provide an opportunity to provide education related to maintaining oral health such as –

brushing teeth twice a day,
use of toothpaste,
flossing and the benefits of gum health for teeth minimising sugary drinks,
keeping a healthy diet, and
options for regular oral health checks via a dental practitioner such as dentist or a dental hygienist.

While cost for dental practitioners may be prohibitive for people identification of early oral problems may offer a means of prevention of severe oral problems.

Conclusion

Oral health in mental health settings is usually a low priority. This is due in the main to competing priorities in the clinical care of people who use specialist areas when the principal specialist health issue is primary, when there exist knowledge gaps, avoidant behaviours of consumers and stigma related to poor oral hygiene and/or mental health. However, cost effective strategies can be used in clinical practice in any setting that can improve the person's oral hygiene (brushing teeth and flossing) and timely referral to oral practitioners such as oral hygienist can improve oral health. Oral assessment tools are also available for clinical staff to use and these range from the complex to the simple to use. Improving physical condition can positively impact on an individual's mental wellbeing, including care for oral health.

Useful Websites

The burden of oral disease available at http://www.cdc.gov/chronicdisease/resources/publications/aag/doh.htm

Caring for my teeth available at http://www.dentalhealth.org/tell-me-about/topic/caring-for-teeth/caring-for-my-teeth

Impacts on oral health – people living with mental illness available at http://oralhealthplan.com.au/tags/people-living-mental-illness

References

Berry, A., Davidson, P., Masters, J., & Rolls, K. (2007). Systematic literature review of oral hygiene practices for intensive care patients receiving mechanical ventilation. *AmeriCan. J.ournal of Critical Care, 16*(6), 552.

Buunk Werkhoven, Y., Dijkstra, A., Schaub, R., Van Der Schans, C., & Spreen, M. (2010). Oral health related quality of life among imprisoned Dutch forensic psychiatric patients. *Journal of Forensic Nursing, 6*(3), 137-143.

Chalmers, J. M., King, P. L., Spencer, A. J., Wright, F., & Carter, K. D. (2005). The oral health assessment tool—validity and reliability. *Australian Dental Journal, 50*(3), 191-199.

de Oliveira, C., Watt, R., & Hamer, M. (2010). Toothbrushing, inflammation, and risk of cardiovascular disease: results from Scottish Health Survey. *British Medical Journal, 340*(may27 1), c2451.

Edward, K.-l., Hemingway, S., & Stephenson, J. (2012). Oral health–a key assessment skill for mental health nurses: a pilot evaluation of an educational intervention. *Mental Health Nursing, 32*(6), 12-16.

Edward, K., Felstead, B. M., & Mahoney, A. M. (2012). Hospitalized mental health patients and oral health. *Journal of Psychiatric & Mental Health Nursing, 19*(5), 419-425.

Eilers, J., Berger, A., & Petersen, M. (1987). *Development, testing, and application of the oral assessment guide.* Paper presented at the Oncology nursing forum.

Eilers, J., & Epstein, J. B. (2004). *Assessment and measurement of oral mucositis.* Paper presented at the Seminars in oncology Nursing.

Fisher, M. A., Borgnakke, W. S., & Taylor, G. W. (2010). Periodontal disease as a risk marker in coronary heart disease and chronic kidney disease. *Current Opinion in Nephrology and Hypertension, 19*(6), 519.

Mori, H., Hirasawa, H., Oda, S., Shiga, H., Matsuda, K., & Nakamura, M. (2006). Oral care reduces incidence of ventilator-associated pneumonia in ICU populations. *Intensive care medicine, 32*(2), 230-236.

Paju, S., & Scannapieco, F. A. (2007). Oral biofilms, periodontitis, and pulmonary infections. *Oral diseases, 13*(6), 508-512.

Persson, K., Axtelius, B., Söderfeldt, B., & Östman, M. (2009). Monitoring oral health and dental attendance in an outpatient psychiatric population. *Journal of Psychiatric and Mental Health Nursing, 16*(3), 263-271.

Ponizovsky, A., M, Zusman, S., P, & Grinshpoon, A. (2009). Oral Health and Hygiene Among Persons With Severe Mental Illness: Reply. *Psychiatric Services, 60*(10), 1402.

Prince, M., Patel, V., Saxena, S., Maj, M., Maselko, J., Phillips, M., & Rahman, A. (2007). No health without mental health. *The Lancet, 370*(9590), 859-877.

Robson, D., & Gray, R. (2007). Serious mental illness and physical health problems: a discussion paper. *International Journal Of Nursing Studies, 44*(3), 457-466.

Salamone, K., Yacoub, E., Mahoney, A.-M., & Edward, K.-l. (2013). Oral Care of Hospitalised Older Patients in the Acute Medical Setting. *Nursing Research and Practice, 2013.*

Stevens, T., Spoors, J., Hale, R., & Bembridge, H. (2010). Perceived oral health needs in psychiatric in-patients: impact of a dedicated dental clinic. *Psychiatric Bulletin, 34*(12), 518.

WHO. (2008). The global burden of disease: 2004 update. In W. H. Organisation (Ed.). Geneva: World Health Organisation.

In: Oral Health
Editor: Julia Renee Barnes

ISBN: 978-1-63482-832-1

Chapter VI

Oral Health: Social Determinants, Role of Nutrition and Impact on Quality of Life Determinants of Oral Health and Quality of Life of Schizophrenic Patients

Frédéric Denis[1*], DDS, MSC, and Benoit Trojak[2], MD, PhD

[1]La Chartreuse Psychiatric Center, Dijon, France
University Hospital of Besançon, Besançon, France
EA 481, Laboratory of Integrative and Clinical Neurosciences, Besançon, France
[2]Department of psychiatry and addictology University Hospital of Dijon, Dijon, France

Abstract

Schizophrenia is a severe mental disorder. It is a ubiquitous disease affecting 1% of the world population. Delusions and hallucinations are symptoms of the disease, but discordance and negation of the body mean these people are not always able to make the right decisions to take care of their health. This is one reason why dental health indicators are very high compared to the general population. Poor oral health is one of the causes of stigma from which these people suffer greatly.

Determinants of the oral health of these patients are multiple. The neurological effects of first-generation antipsychotic drugs are multiple (dyskinesia, extrapyramidal syndrome, myasthenia gravis, and trismus) and disrupt the motricity of the oral region. The metabolic effects of second-generation antipsychotic drugs (dyslipidemia, hyperglycemia, weight gain, hyperprolactinemia, and cardiovascular ischemic disorders)

[*] frederic.denis@chs-chartreuse.fr.

and more generally anti-cholinergic pharmacopoeia worsen dental problems further. There are also other determinants of oral health of schizophrenic patients, such as disruption of the nociceptive pathways, taking psychoactive substances, smoking, poor diet and lifestyle, and lower socioeconomic status. The lack of somatic care in relation to the division between body and mind must also be mentioned. Lastly, health promotion activities are inadequate for these populations and health professionals lack training in this area.

Studies on the subject are difficult to implement because patients do not readily consent to the exploration of an organ with a strong symbolic and emotional component. Studies that target only schizophrenic patients are few and far between and only concern hospitalized patients, i.e. few patients. The state of knowledge in this area has a low level of evidence. Outstanding issues are numerous regarding the effectiveness of preventive actions and management of patients with very specific needs. In this context, we analyzed the impact of poor oral health of schizophrenic patients on their overall health and quality of life through motivational and cognitive constraints imposed by the symptoms of schizophrenia, but also through the unique perspective of caregivers and society about this disease that is too often stigmatized.

Introduction

Schizophrenia is a ubiquitous disease that affects 1% of the world population [1]. This is a severe mental disorder characterized by a diverse set of symptoms of varying intensity: the most impressive are delusions, hallucinations, and mental dissociation and for the most disabling of them, and also social withdrawal, negation of the body and cognitive difficulties [2]. In essence, schizophrenic patients are not always able to perceive their health problems and / or make the right decisions to solve them autonomously [3]. This results in the coexistence of psychiatric disorders and many organic comorbidities [4-6]. Two-way relationships are clearly established: mental illness that causes organic diseases and organic diseases that can be complicated by psychiatric disorders. Thus, among the usual somatic comorbidities of these patients, we mention, metabolic disorders or "metabolic syndrome" (diabetes, hypertension, dyslipidemia, and abdominal obesity), malnutrition, poor lifestyle, and poor oral health [5, 7-10]. The latter is often found by carers. It is one of the causes of stigma cruelly suffered by these patients (2). Also, antipsychotic medications have side effects that are combined with all the co-morbidities to which they are exposed [11]. This is one of the reasons why schizophrenic patients have a lower life expectancy of 15 to 20 years compared to the general population, with the exception of suicide [12]. Improving the management of somatic disorders is therefore a major public health issue.

1. Schizophrenia

Schizophrenia is a serious mental disorder, chronic and complex, whose occurrence depends on the presence of genetic and environmental factors. It affects around 0.7% to 1% of the world population [1]. It occurs in all regions of the world, but is more frequent in urban areas and among migrants, most often between 15 and 25 years. In humans, schizophrenia symptoms typically begin in adolescence around 15-16 years; in women a little later at the age of 20 or early 30s [13, 14]. The diagnosis of schizophrenia can be defined from the description of the symptoms of the *Diagnostic and Statistical Manual of Mental Disorders* (DSM-V; 5th revised edition), a work that is the subject of broad consensus [15]. Schizophrenia is characterized by a break in contact with the surrounding world, withdrawal from reality, and autistic thinking. Specifically, there is a disruption of the usual balance of emotions and thoughts. This severe mental illness is characterized by many symptoms, which can vary from one person to another and are not always present at the same time. They are classified into three categories:

Positive symptoms consist of abnormally active productions of the mind, such as hallucinations, delusions, thought disorders, and behavioral disorders.

Negative symptoms correspond to a decrease or lack of reaction or the usual response to a given situation. The patient spends a lot of time in bed, is unwilling to participate in daily tasks, and is limited to basic needs (food, sleep, etc.). The warning signs of these symptoms are social withdrawal, lack of energy and motivation, reduced emotional expression, or expression of ideas.

Cognitive symptoms affect the person's ability to understand, analyze, and remember information. The person has difficulty concentrating or staying focused on a specific task. Short-term memory can be affected and the patient often finds difficulties in implementing activities in their daily lives (medication and personal and dental hygiene). The schizophrenic is ambivalent, disinterested in the surroundings, and has difficulty making decisions. This is in association with social dysfunction, ambivalence, loss of control, and attention and memory problems that interfere with learning in some individuals [16].

Causes

Research has highlighted that there is not just one simple cause, but rather several important variables factors that interact with each other to cause the disease and its relapses. Interaction between biological and environmental factors contributes to the disease. Among the biological factors that appear to contribute to schizophrenia are the recurrence of the disease in the family, brain abnormalities, neuropsychological fragility, biological disturbances of brain neurotransmitter (serotonin and dopamine), etc. Environmental causes include emotional upheaval, professional or academic pressures related to performance, inadequate social support, negative emotions expressed by the entourage (hostile, intrusive attitude, and aggressiveness), alcohol and drug abuse issues, etc. It is important to note that many people suffer such stress on a daily basis; however, they will not develop schizophrenia if there are no biological predisposing factors for this disease [17].

Treatment

Treatment of schizophrenia is based on antipsychotic drugs combined with various psychotherapeutic modalities, including rehabilitation and reintegration programs. These programs are intended to help the person with schizophrenia to reintegrate into professional and social life. The aim is to overcome the deficits and disabilities caused by the disease and allow patients to maintain their identity, dignity, and self-esteem [18].

Schizophrenia and Mortality

Mortality of schizophrenic patients is 4.5 times higher than in the general population for all ages, sexes, and causes (natural or not) [16]. The leading cause of death among schizophrenic patients is suicide (4.2%) followed by cancer pathologies (2.2%), particularly breast cancer in women and lung cancer in men, and cardiovascular disease (2%). The mortality rate by "natural" causes is 2.5 times higher than in the general population; life expectancy is reduced by 20% [20]. However, premature death from "natural" causes seems linked to the adverse lifestyles of patients and associated factors, such as exposure to tobacco, alcohol, psychoactive substances, poor social conditions, and adverse effects of antipsychotic treatment (metabolic syndrome, cardiovascular disease, etc.) [12].

2. Co-Morbidities Frequently Associated with Schizophrenia and Adverse Effects of Antipsychotic Drugs

2.1. Schizophrenia and Cardiovascular Disease

Risk Factors

In schizophrenic patients, the prevalence of risk factors for cardiovascular disease is higher than in the general population: [21]

- Obesity: 42% of schizophrenic patients of the US population have a body mass index (BMI) greater than or equal to 27 compared to 27% for patients from the same population
- Smoking: the prevalence is 75%, compared to 25% in the general population
- Diabetes: the prevalence is 13% compared to 3% in the general population
- High blood pressure (hypertension): affects 27% against 17% in the general population
- Physical inactivity
- Hypercholesterolemia

The risk of coronary heart disease is between 2 and 3.6 times higher in schizophrenic patients compared to the general population [22].

Coronary Heart Disease

A correlation exists between antipsychotic drugs and an increased fluctuation in blood pressure [22]. Studies also show that antipsychotic factors contribute to cardiovascular risks, such as obesity, dyslipidemia, diabetes, and hypertension. In addition, some treatments (olanzapine) have a greater impact on the risk of developing coronary artery disease at 10 years compared to other atypical antipsychotic drugs [22].

Ventricular Arrhythmias and Prolongation of the QTc Interval

All antipsychotic drugs can generate prolongation of ventricular repolarization, signaled by a prolongation of the QTc interval on the electrocardiogram (ECG). This conduction disorder runs the risk of torsades de pointes as ventricular arrhythmias may be complicated by ventricular fibrillation and risk of sudden death [23].

Myocarditis

Several case studies have reported the occurrence of myocarditis under clozapine [24]. Although infrequent, it is potentially fatal in 10% of cases. Myocarditis consecutive to treatment with clozapine exposes the risk of developing cardiomyopathy after approximately 6-8 months of treatment with this molecule [24].

2.2. Schizophrenia and Addictive Behavior

Severe mental disorders like schizophrenia generate significant suffering. The simultaneous use of alcohol or drugs (cannabis, tobacco, etc.) is common [25]. The subjects seek in these consumptions easing of mental disorders, stimulation of intellectual capacity, and improved negative symptoms. Comorbidities caused by addictive behaviors are numerous (neuronal degeneration, and liver, pancreatic, dental, and periodontal problems, etc.) related to the toxicity of the substances used [10, 26]. The percentage of smokers in the population of schizophrenic patients is twice that of smokers in the general population and consumption is often greater. Furthermore, the presence of addiction associated with schizophrenia increases the risk of hetero-aggressive violence [27].

2.3. Schizophrenia and Metabolic Syndrome

Metabolic syndrome is defined by a combination of carbohydrate, vascular, and lipid disorders or is associated with being overweight. Combinations of the metabolic disorders may act synergistically in the body and cause type 2 diabetes, predisposing the patient to the risk of atherosclerosis and potential complications.

Table 1. Definition of metabolic syndrome according to the International Diabetes Federation

Overweight	
Waist size greater than or equal to 102 cm for Eurasian males and 88 cm for females	
Mandatory criterion	
At least two of the following four parameters:	
Triglycerides > 150mg / dl or current specific treatment	
HDL < 40 mg / dL in males and < 50 mg / dL in females or current specific treatment	
Blood pressure:	≥ 130 mmHg systolic and
	≥ 85 mmHg diastolic
Or current specific treatment	
Hyperglycemia > 100 mg / dl or current specific treatment for type 2 diabetes	

This is not in itself a disease entity, but a set of clinical and biological disturbances easy to diagnose in daily practice. There are many definitions of this syndrome. We retain that of the International Diabetes Federation (Table 1). Schizophrenics are more likely to have metabolic syndrome. The risk of metabolic syndrome varies with the antipsychotic molecule used to treat the patient [5] (Table 2).

2.4. Schizophrenia and Glycemic Control Disorder

Antipsychotic drugs act on the metabolism of glucose and insulin. They may cause diabetes. Second-generation antipsychotic drugs (APIIG) have a 1.3 times higher risk of causing diabetes than first-generation antipsychotic drugs (API) [28]. The risk of developing diabetes in APIIG is also linked to being overweight. The prevalence of type 2 diabetes in schizophrenic patients is 2-3 times higher than in the general population [29]. Predisposition to a malfunction of the insulin-glucose homeostasis exists even in patients not treated with antipsychotic drugs [30]. Schizophrenia would thus be an independent risk factor for the development of diabetes [30]. In this case, even controlling the behavioral and physiological risk factors involved in diabetes, genetic factors involved in schizophrenia may influence metabolic control [29, 30].

Table 2. Risk of developing the metabolic syndrome according to the antipsychotic drug (adapted from De Hert et al., 2011) [45]

Treatment	Risk of metabolic syndrome
Chlorpromazine (CN)	High (limited data)
Clozapine (CN)	High
Olanzapine	High
Quetiapine (APA)	Moderate
Amisulpride (CN)	Average
Risperidone (APA)	Average
Aripiprazole (APA)	Low
Haloperidol (CN)	Low

CN: conventional neuroleptics, APA: Atypical antipsychotics.

2.5. Schizophrenia and Dyslipidemia

Antipsychotic treatment may induce a decrease in HDL-cholesterol, and an increase in LDL cholesterol, total cholesterol, and triglycerides [22]. The risk of dyslipidemia is higher in descending order with olanzapine, clozapine, and quetapine than with risperidone and aripiprazole [31].

2.6. Obesity and Schizophrenia

Schizophrenics are 2.8 to 3.5 times more likely to become obese [32]. The risk of weight gain in APIIG or APIG affects between 15% and 72% of patients [29]. The risk of weight gain with antipsychotic drugs corresponds to neurobiological mechanisms. Among the assumptions, a change in affinity to receptors promoting weight gain (H1, 5HT2C, and D2), influences the hormones regulating appetite, diet, and lifestyle factors, and increases appetite and / or food intake [33].

2.7. Schizophrenia and Osteoporosis

A decrease in bone mineral density in schizophrenic patients is observed compared to controls of about 40% and 72% according to studies [10, 34] and leads to a higher risk of fracture [35].

The risk factors are:

- High levels of prolactin
- Physical inactivity
- Smoking, alcohol, and drugs
- Diet deficient in vitamins
- Decreased sun exposure
- Polydipsia

2.8. Schizophrenia and Respiratory Diseases

An increased incidence of death by suffocation has been described. It is linked to tardive dyskinesia, tachyphagies, or false routes [36]. A high frequency of obstructive sleep apnea occurs of which one of the causes is obesity [37]. Finally, there is a higher prevalence of angina and respiratory symptoms and altered respiratory function compared to the general population [38, 39].

2.9. Schizophrenia and Cancers

Studies on the prevalence of cancer in schizophrenics are conflicting. For breast cancer, 13 studies conducted between 1986 and 2008 and involving more than 6000 patients showed different results ranging from a 52% increase to a 40% decrease of cancers observed [40]. For lung cancer, several studies report an increased risk [41, 42] while others contradicted these data [43]. The results for digestive cancers are similar [43, 44]. However, no studies have identified on the prevalence of oral cavity cancers in schizophrenic patients.

2.10. Schizophrenia and Neurological Disorders

APIG are more often the cause of extrapyramidal disorders than APIIG. Their occurrence is associated with the affinity of D2 dopamine receptors; 5-HT 2A serotonin is dose dependent [45]. Tardive dyskinesia is predominantly orofacial (dystonia, dyskinesia, stereotyping, etc.), but sometimes affect other parts of the body in the form of uncontrollable movements of the legs (akathisia). These disturbances persist even after discontinuation of treatment [46].

2.11. Schizophrenia and Hematological Disorders

The risk of hematologic disorders such as neutropenia by agranulocytosis under clozapine is well documented. Agranulocytosis is lethal in 5% to 10% of cases. Other antipsychotic drugs are either devoid of possible hematologic complications of the leukocyte lineage [47].

2.12. Schizophrenia and Exposure to HIV, HCV, HBV, and Tuberculosis

The prevalence of hepatitis C in patients with psychiatric disorders is between 6.8% and 8.5%, i.e. much higher values than in the general population, particularly in France [48, 49]. The prevalence of HIV and tuberculosis is also higher. This is explained by overexposure by risky sexual behavior with multiple partners and the use of alcohol and drugs with multiple partners [50].

2.13. Schizophrenia and Immune Weakness

The set of co-morbid disorders suffered by these patients, i.e. the metabolic syndrome, nutritional deficiencies, non-compliance with lifestyle and dietary rules, treatment side effects (neutropenia with agranulocytosis), addictive behavior (alcohol, drugs, etc.), smoking, risky behavior, over-exposure to HIV and HCV, and insecurity, means that these patients are predisposed to immune weakness [51, 52].

2.14. Schizophrenia and Violence

Hetero-aggressive risk is attributable to addictive disorders more than mental disorders [53]. The increased risk of violence is higher among schizophrenic women than men and the risk of being arrested for violence is 23 times higher in women, whereas it is 4.6 times in men compared to the general population [54].

2.15. Schizophrenia and Pain

For a long time it was considered that schizophrenic patients were insensitive to pain. Recent studies have shown that this is not the case [55]. Diagnostic delays are sometimes observed related to, firstly, confusion in reading the pain signs that are clouded by the symptoms of schizophrenia and, secondly, the lack of verbalization of pain by the patient.

This lack of response is due to indifference to pain rather than insensitivity [56]. In this case, it often leads to "somatic disorders" indifference by patients and to detrimental treatment delays for the patient [57].

2.16. Schizophrenia and a Lifestyle Unfavorable to Health

The main causes of mortality are of cardiovascular somatic origin. Factors influencing this mortality are related to lifestyle caused by the psychiatric pathology. It leads to an unhealthy lifestyle (diet rich in carbohydrates, low in vegetables and fish, physical inactivity, and smoking), negation of the body (neglect of personal hygiene and lack of exercise), and risky behavior (drugs and alcoholism). There are also side effects of psychotropic medication of which patients are misinformed by caregivers, insecurity, difficulty for them to invest in the preservation of their physical health, and poor capacity to respond to care systems in general for their specific needs [45, 58].

3. Schizophrenia and Oral Health

Excessive consumption of alcohol, smoking, and poor eating habits can affect oral health. These behaviors may contribute to the development of caries and infectious periodontal disease (dental plaque) [59]. Social, environmental factors, and lifestyle, especially marginalization, are also factors of poor oral health [60]. In the absence of treatment, they lead to early tooth loss. Frequent consumption of sugary drinks and foods and inadequate fluoride exposure increase the risk of caries. Smoking, diabetes, and immune deficiency mainly contribute to periodontal disease [60, 61]. Oral health is an important determinant of the quality of life and overall health [62, 63].

In this area, research in recent years has focused mainly on the possible repercussions of oral disorders on the health of individuals and the manifestations of general diseases in the oral sphere. The existence of a relationship between metabolic disorders and oral infectious diseases has gradually imposed firstly with the evolution of knowledge on the pathophysiology of metabolic syndrome, and secondly by finding that certain oral sphere infectious diseases, such as periodontal disease, had already been associated with each of the metabolic syndrome components (periodontal disease and diabetes, periodontal disease and cardiovascular disease, tooth loss and obesity, etc.) in the general population [64, 68].

3.1. Epidemiology

Studies on oral health determinants of mental health patients are relatively common, except those related to schizophrenia. A literature search using PubMed data / Medline, with the keywords “schizophrenia,” “dental status,” and “oral health surveys” in the period from 2000 to 2014 returns 10 studies related to oral health schizophrenic patients. These studies were performed in nine different countries (Spain, People's Republic of China, Turkey, United Kingdom, Denmark, Israel, Iran, India, and Japan).

Table 3. Literature review

Study	Year	Country	Outpatients or hospitalized patients	N	Average age	DMF (1)	Periodontal indices	Other
McCreadie et al.,[78]	2004	UK	Outpatient	428	43	____	____	Associated variables studies
Chu et al.,[75]	2010	Taiwan	Hospitalized	1103	50.8	13.9	____	Associated variables studies
Arnaiz et al.,[69]	2011	Spain	Outpatient	66 schizophrenic patients66 control patients	40	DMF: 13.51DMF: 7.80	2.321.04	PANSS-P (2) correlated with lower DMFT
Chu et al.,[74]	2011	Taiwan	Hospitalized	878	50.6	13.9	____	BMI (3): 24.7
Nielsen et al.,[77]	2011	Denmark	Outpatient	21 417 for 200618 892 between 2004 and 2006	42.5341.7 0	____	____	correlated with lower DMFT
Chu et al., [70]	2012	Taiwan	Hospitalized	1103	50.8	13.9	35.9% CPI(4) ≥ 3vs. 5% control	____
Tani et al.,[76]	2012	Japan	Hospitalized	523	55.6	18.8 for 40-59 years	____	Associated variables studies
Eltas et al.,[71]	2013	Turkey	Outpatient	33 patients with hypo salivation-inducing medication	31.8	8.4	PI(5) 80% ±39 BP(6) 73%± 32	Salivary flow 0.23ml/mn
				20 patients with hyper salivation-inducing medication		8.2	PI 58± 41 BP 49±37	1.12ml/mn
Nikfarjam et al., [72]	2013	Iran	Hospitalized	123	38.81	19.43	____	PANSS-N correlated with higher DMF
Chu et al.,[73]	2013	Taiwan	Hospitalized	1103	50.8	____	____	37.5% needed fixed prostheses and 65% needed dentures

1-DMF: Decay, Missing, Filled.
2-PANSS: Positive and Negative Syndrome Scale.
3-BMI: Body Mass Index.
4-CPI: Community Periodontal Index.
4-PI: Papillary index.
5-BI: Blending index.

Analysis of these data was performed using two indices, the DMF (Decay, Missing, Filled) and the CPI index (Community Periodontal Index) (Table 3).

The DMF reference index was used to evaluate dental health. It assesses the carious pathology. The CPI index measures the oral hygiene status and periodontal disease through evaluation of three parameters (bleeding, subgingival plaque, and periodontal pocket). The CPI index is the reference index of the World Health Organization (WHO).

For the DMF

Analysis of publications shows that the DMF is twice higher in schizophrenic patients compared to a matched control group. Arniaz et al., (2011) compared the DMF index and CPI of a group of 66 patients followed up as outpatients with a matched group of the general population. They found a DMF of 13.51 vs. 7.27, respectively [69]. In another study of 1108 hospitalized subjects, Chu et al., (2012) found a DMF of 13.94 vs. 8.39 for their control group of 2660 subjects [70].

The number of missing teeth is high compared to the number of treated teeth, and the need for functional rehabilitation (denture or fixed) is significant in relation to the need of the general population [69, 71, 72]. Chu et al., (2013) reported three factors favorable to rehabilitation with a removable prosthesis for psychiatric patients: a low level of education, length of stay, and age [73]. Chu et al., (2011) showed that of 1103 schizophrenic patients, 37% needed a fixed prosthesis and 63% needed a removable prosthesis [74].

For the CPI

The CPI is twice that observed in a control group and is high compared to the general population [69, 70]. Arnaiz et al., found a CPI of 2.32 in patients followed up as outpatients against 1.04 in a matched control group [69]. 90.7% of the hospitalized schizophrenic patients studied by Chu et al., (2012) had a CPI $\geq$ 2 [70]. This means that most patients with schizophrenia have a need for periodontal care (learn hygiene and scaling). Eltas et al., (2012) showed that the periodontal status changed by the absorption of antipsychotic drugs. This study involved two matched groups of patients: the first group took medication causing xerostomia (risperidone, quetiapine, and olanzapine); the second group took drugs stimulating the salivary flow (clozapine). Periodontal health was more degraded in the first group with more bleeding on probing and plaque. The small amount of saliva correlated with a high plaque index and bleeding index [71].

Chu et al., (2011) studied the relationship between body mass index and the risk of caries in schizophrenic patients treated with APIIG. They found no relationship between treatment with antipsychotic drugs and oral condition. However, taking into account the patient's age, they showed that the oral condition deteriorated in the leanest and eldest patients [74].

Scientists have studied the relationship between negative and positive symptoms of schizophrenia assessed by the PANSS (Positive and Negative Syndrome Scale) and oral health. They noticed that patients with higher negative symptoms and a high DMF had a greater number of missing and decayed teeth compared to patients with positive symptoms. The results were similar with the need for periodontal care; patients with high negative PANSS had more need for care than the others [69, 71, 72, 75].

More generally, all studies agree on the need to care for these populations, which in addition to limited financial resources and limited access to health systems, frequently smoke and present side effects of antipsychotic treatments. All authors agree on the need to build specific prevention programs related to the needs of these populations [72, 75-78]. However, the results of these studies are limited because the populations studied are often hospitalized patients who are in acute decompensation of the disease or are too deficient. We can therefore assume that the data collected only partially reflect the oral health status of these populations. In France, only 20% of the population suffering from schizophrenia is hospitalized [79]. Moreover, in all studies, patients were included without selection, which induces an obvious bias. We can assume for example that patients who are not willing to participate in these studies are likely to be reluctant to have a dental checkup because of their poor oral health. In this case, the real DMF and CPI score in schizophrenic patients would be higher than the results announced.

3.2. Difficulties of Good Oral Health of Schizophrenic Patients

3.2.1. Impact of Mental Illness

The symptoms of schizophrenia reduce the planning and implementation capacity of the hygienic procedures of everyday life, such as oral hygiene.

These disorders result from a disturbance in executive functions. We also note that the default context analysis and reasoning errors associated with cognitive impairment cause patients not to perceive the importance of their health problems and not to take appropriate decisions to resolve them [80, 81]. In this context, 60% of schizophrenic patients do not perceive their problems and are not motivated seek care or even oppose it [82]. In general, the disruption of the train of thought related to mental illness is that patients do not perceive these needs and are therefore slow to consult. In this case, it is important to anticipate in order to identify health problems because the intensity of cognitive disorders correlates with lack of initiative [83]. This problem is even more important than the learning capacity of the population. Several studies have shown the effectiveness of the principles of "social skills training" in improving adherence to therapeutic treatments and improving social skills in schizophrenic patients (skills at work, social functioning, etc.) [84]. Ponizovsky et al., (2009) saw an improvement of the oral health status of hospitalized patients undergoing regular dental follow-up by benefitting all patients hospitalized for more than year from regular monitoring by a dentist [85].

3.2.2. Weight of Iatrogenic Factors (Table 4)

- The link between periodontal disease and metabolic syndrome is unclear. It follows from the combination of an imbalance of intracellular oxidative mechanisms with an increase of inflammatory mechanisms related to metabolic dysfunction. Insulin resistance is a consequence of disturbances of oxidative mechanisms, which can be improved or aggravated by factors such as smoking, alcohol, age, diet, physical activity, and socio-economic level [64, 67, 68]. Studies should explore the nature of this link with schizophrenic patients with significant metabolic deregulation [21].
- First-generation antipsychotic-induced extra pyramidal syndrome (inhibition of dopamine D2 receptors and serotonin 5HT2A) disturbs the dexterity required to achieve effective brushing and it manifests at the orofacial level by dystonias and

dyskinesias that disrupt the oral function, such as phonation and deglutition [86]. We distinguish acute dystonia manifested by the contraction of the muscles of the neck, face, throat, and eyes. The mandible can be locked in the open position with protrusive tongue or on locked in the closed position (lockjaw) with retrusive tongue. Moreover, airways are sometimes blocked by laryngospasm and a swollen tongue. The second side effect is pseudo-parkinsonian symptoms: antipsychotic drugs can cause a decrease in blinking of the eyes, drooling, and monotonous speech [87].

- Dry mouth induced by antipsychotic drugs (Table 4) favors the occurrence of caries, gingivitis, and periodontal disease. This factor added to others, such as poor oral and food hygiene, smoking, and poor dental monitoring, contributes to poor oral health in schizophrenic patients [76].
- Salivation induced by antipsychotic drugs, such as clozapine, promotes perlèche and drooling. Parotitis is also seen under clozapine [88].

Table 4. Main side effects of drugs used in mental health that affect oral health according to the *British Society for Disability and Oral Health* [94]

	Xerostomia	Drowsiness	Agranulo cytosis	Tardive dyskinesia	Tremor	syncope	Hypo-tension	Thrombo cytopenia	Immuno suppression	Apathy
Amitryptiline	■						■	■	■	
Benzo diazépine	■	■					■			
Cannabis	■									
Chlorpro mazine	■	■					■			■
Chlordiaze poxide		■								
Dexamphe tamine sulfate	■				■					
Clozapine	Hypersalivation		■	■						
Dothiepin	■									
Fluphenazine deconate	■	■		■						
Fluoxetine										Aggression
Haloperidole	■	■								
Lithium carbonate					■	■				
Lofepramine	■			■	■					
Methylphen idate hydrochloride	■				■			■		
Mono-amine Oxidase inihibitors	■						■	■	■	
Prochlorpe razine	■	■		■			■			
Procyclidine	■	■								
Promazine hydrochloride	■	■								■
Risperidone	■	■								■
Thioridazine	■	■								■

3.2.4. Insufficient Dental Care Management: Reasons

- The mouth is an intimate part of the body, full of symbolism and representation and to which access is difficult for caregivers because of the symptoms of the disease. This is an area of little investment by professionals. Moreover, prevention and promotion programs based on knowledge of the general population have not proven to be highly effective once transposed to patients with severe psychiatric disorders [4, 89].
- Early detection is important to identify health problems. Indeed, the lack of initiative is correlated with the severity of cognitive impairment. The sickest patients do not seek treatment voluntarily and will have little incentive to change their behavior in order to have a healthy lifestyle and good oral hygiene [90].
- Professionals are adverse to caring for these patients (fear of mental illness, lack of training) and patients to the health care system in general (difficult access to the district environment, cost, etc.), which are additional barriers to somatic care. Finally, misuse of the care system is detected in these patients, explaining the late appearance at consultations, and lack of visits and follow-up: this may be due to apathy, poor initiative, and repeated forgetfulness by these patients. The executive functions disorder may partly explain the difficulty these patients have to get to a given place at a given time. Other symptoms such as anxiety, phobia of transport, or limited financial resources are factors that contribute to the lack of access to the health care system.
- Finally, the overall approach to mental health patients is rarely included in institutional care projects. But the obvious link between metabolic disturbance, oral health, and schizophrenia should guide practices toward comprehensive care including nutrition, diabetic control, monitoring of cardiovascular disorders, and the concerted effort of care teams.

4. Oral Disease Management

The Cochrane review (Khokhar et al., 2011) aimed to identify studies with a high level of evidence of effective oral health tips for improving the quality of oral health of schizophrenic patients. The authors of the review note that there is no high-level evidence study to support the direction of current practices [91]. Thus, the recommendations for practice of the "British Society for Disability and Oral Health" are therefore based on expert consensus. But in the light of this report, the co-occurrences between oral disease, schizophrenia, and the somatic disorders associated with it are many. Improving oral health concerns improving overall health and vice versa. In this context, it is important to consider comprehensive care management. Indeed, poor diet, smoking, and drug interactions can lead to loss of nutritional intake and be an aggravating factor of periodontal disease [92]. It is also important to consider lifestyle because it is possible to prevent and treat a set of individual (brushing motivation), community (destigmatization), and professional (personal training) measures. This is an area of action with often little investment due to a sense of powerlessness to act on these factors. However, there are studies showing that it is possible to intervene successfully on some of these determinants, seeking the collaboration of patient care programs through motivational approaches [93, 85] They address how to help patients manage their smoking, a sedentary lifestyle, their dietary imbalances, and their dental hygiene. The identification of somatic problems where patients live, especially when living in a community, is also essential. For this, it is necessary to train people that may frequently interact with patients, especially the family environment, social services, and medical workers, district nurses, and GPs.

Conclusion

Studies show that patients with severe mental disorders have many somatic comorbidities and a life expectancy of 15 to 20 years less than in the general population. Oral health, although often overlooked, is intimately linked to these somatic comorbidities, which also shares many risk factors. It therefore appears obvious to act simultaneously on these common risk factors in order to improve overall health and therefore oral health. However, unlike the general population where prevention programs have proven effective in patients with severe mental disorders, the mechanisms of motivation and identification needs are different. Oral health assessment tools adapted to these populations remain to be developed. Moreover, research is required to specify the type of prevention and promotion programs tailored to the specific needs of these populations.

References

[1] Esan OB, Ojagbemi A, Gureje O. Epidemiology of schizophrenia--an update with a focus on developing countries. *Int. Rev. Psychiatry Abingdon Engl.* oct 2012; 24(5):387-92.

[2] Ling Y, Watanabe M, Yoshii H, Akazawa K. Characteristics linked to the reduction of stigma towards schizophrenia: a pre-and-post study of parents of adolescents attending an educational program. *BMC Public Health.* 2014;14:258.

[3] Grisso T, Appelbaum PS. Comparison of standards for assessing patients' capacities to make treatment decisions. *Am. J. Psychiatry. juill* 1995;152(7):1033-7.

[4] Tosh G, Clifton A, Bachner M. *General Physical Health Advice for People with Serious Mental Illness.* Schizophr Bull [Internet]. 7 janv 2011 [cité 12 janv 2015];37(4):671-3. Disponible sur: http://schizophreniabulletin.oxfordjournals.org/content/37/4/671

[5] De Hert M, van Winkel R, Van Eyck D, Hanssens L, Wampers M, Scheen A, et al., Prevalence of diabetes, metabolic syndrome and metabolic abnormalities in schizophrenia over the course of the illness: a cross-sectional study. *Clin. Pract. Epidemiol. Ment. Health CP EMH.* 2006;2:14.

[6] Wildgust HJ, Hodgson R, Beary M. The paradox of premature mortality in schizophrenia: new research questions. *J. Psychopharmacol. Oxf. Engl.* nov 2010;24(4 Suppl):9-15.

[7] Cohn T, Prud'homme D, Streiner D, Kameh H, Remington G. Characterizing coronary heart disease risk in chronic schizophrenia: high prevalence of the metabolic syndrome. *Can. J. Psychiatry Rev. Can. Psychiatr.* nov 2004;49(11):753-60.

[8] Angelillo IF, Nobile CG, Pavia M, De Fazio P, Puca M, Amati A. Dental health and treatment needs in institutionalized psychiatric patients in Italy. *Community Dent Oral Epidemiol.* déc 1995;23(6):360-4.

[9] Friedlander AH, Friedlander IK, Eth S, Freymiller EG. Dental management of child and adolescent patients with schizophrenia. *ASDC J. Dent Child.* oct 1993;60(4-5):281-7.

[10] Leucht S, Burkard T, Henderson J, Maj M, Sartorius N. Physical illness and schizophrenia: a review of the literature. *Acta Psychiatr Scand.* nov 2007;116(5):317-33.

[11] Joukamaa M, Heliövaara M, Knekt P, Aromaa A, Raitasalo R, Lehtinen V. Schizophrenia, neuroleptic medication and mortality. *Br. J. Psychiatry J. Ment Sci.* févr 2006;188:122-7.

[12] Pack S. Poor physical health and mortality in patients with schizophrenia. *Nurs Stand R Coll Nurs G B* 1987. 28 févr 2009;23(21):41-5.

[13] Häfner H, an der Heiden W. Epidemiology of schizophrenia. *Can. J. Psychiatry Rev. Can Psychiatr.* mars 1997;42(2):139-51.

[14] Schizophrénie [Internet]. [cité 2 janv 2015]. Disponible sur: http://www.inserm.fr/thematiques/neurosciences-sciences-cognitives-neurologie-psychiatrie/dossiers-d-information/schizophrenie

[15] DSM-5 | psychiatry.org [Internet]. [cité 20 janv 2015]. Disponible sur: http://www.psychiatry.org/dsm5

[16] Nom de la Maladie: Schizophrénie text redigee par - article_llorca_ schizophrenie.pdf [Internet]. [cité 20 janv 2015]. Disponible sur: http://www.fondation-fondamental.org/upload/pdf/ article_llorca_ schizophrenie.pdf

[17] Pearlson GD. Etiologic, Phenomenologic, and Endophenotypic Overlap of Schizophrenia and Bipolar Disorder. *Annu. Rev. Clin. Psychol.* 12 janv 2015;

[18] Gillam T, Williams R. Understanding schizophrenia: a guide for newly qualified nurses. *Br. J. Community Nurs.* févr 2008;13(2):84-8.

[19] Hoang U, Stewart R, Goldacre MJ. Mortality after hospital discharge for people with schizophrenia or bipolar disorder: *retrospective study of linked English hospital episode statistics,* 1999-2006. *BMJ.* 2011;343:d5422.

[20] Tran E, Rouillon F, Loze J-Y, Casadebaig F, Philippe A, Vitry F, et al., Cancer mortality in patients with schizophrenia: an 11-year prospective cohort study. *Cancer.* 1 août 2009;115(15):3555-62.

[21] Goff DC, Sullivan LM, McEvoy JP, Meyer JM, Nasrallah HA, Daumit GL, et al., A comparison of ten-year cardiac risk estimates in schizophrenia patients from the CATIE study and matched controls. *Schizophr Res.* 1 déc 2005;80(1):45-53.

[22] Daumit GL, Goff DC, Meyer JM, Davis VG, Nasrallah HA, McEvoy JP, et al., Antipsychotic effects on estimated 10-year coronary heart disease risk in the CATIE schizophrenia study. *Schizophr Res.* oct 2008;105(1-3):175-87.

[23] Glassman AH, Bigger JT. Antipsychotic drugs: prolonged QTc interval, torsade de pointes, and sudden death. *Am. J. Psychiatry.* nov 2001;158(11):1774-82.

[24] Kontoangelos K, Loizos S, Kanakakis J, Smyrnis N, Economou M, Bergiannaki JD, et al., Myocarditis after administration of clozapine. *Eur. Rev. Med. Pharmacol Sci.* août 2014;18(16):2383-6.

[25] Jané-Llopis E, Matytsina I. Mental health and alcohol, drugs and tobacco: a review of the comorbidity between mental disorders and the use of alcohol, tobacco and illicit drugs. *Drug Alcohol Rev.* nov 2006;25(6):515-36.

[26] Sokal J, Messias E, Dickerson FB, Kreyenbuhl J, Brown CH, Goldberg RW, et al., Comorbidity of medical illnesses among adults with serious mental illness who are receiving community psychiatric services. *J. Nerv Ment Dis. juin* 2004;192(6):421-7.

[27] Ringen PA, Lagerberg TV, Birkenaes AB, Engn J, Faerden A, Jónsdottir H, et al., Differences in prevalence and patterns of substance use in schizophrenia and bipolar disorder. *Psychol. Med.* sept 2008;38(9):1241-9.

[28] Okumura Y, Ito H, Kobayashi M, Mayahara K, Matsumoto Y, Hirakawa J. Prevalence of diabetes and antipsychotic prescription patterns in patients with schizophrenia: a nationwide retrospective cohort study. *Schizophr Res.* juin 2010;119(1-3):145-52.

[29] Newcomer JW, Haupt DW, Fucetola R, Melson AK, Schweiger JA, Cooper BP, et al., Abnormalities in glucose regulation during antipsychotic treatment of schizophrenia. *Arch. Gen. Psychiatry.* avr 2002;59(4):337-45.

[30] Bellivier F. Schizophrenia, antipsychotics and diabetes: Genetic aspects. *Eur. Psychiatry J. Assoc. Eur. Psychiatr.* déc 2005;20 Suppl 4:S335-9.

[31] Rummel-Kluge C, Komossa K, Schwarz S, Hunger H, Schmid F, Lobos CA, et al., Head-to-head comparisons of metabolic side effects of second generation antipsychotics in the treatment of schizophrenia: a systematic review and meta-analysis. *Schizophr Res.* nov 2010;123(2-3):225-33.

[32] DE Hert M, Correll CU, Bobes J, Cetkovich-Bakmas M, Cohen D, Asai I, et al., Physical illness in patients with severe mental disorders. I. Prevalence, impact of medications and disparities in health care. *World Psychiatry Off J. World Psychiatr Assoc WPA.* févr 2011;10(1):52-77.

[33] Balt SL, Galloway GP, Baggott MJ, Schwartz Z, Mendelson J. Mechanisms and genetics of antipsychotic-associated weight gain. *Clin. Pharmacol. Ther.* juill 2011;90(1):179-83.

[34] Meyer JM, Lehman D. Bone mineral density in male schizophrenia patients: a review. *Ann. Clin. Psychiatry Off J. Am. Acad. Clin. Psychiatr. mars* 2006;18(1):43-8.

[35] Graham SM, Howgate D, Anderson W, Howes C, Heliotis M, Mantalaris A, et al., Risk of osteoporosis and fracture incidence in patients on antipsychotic medication. *Expert Opin Drug Saf.* juill 2011;10(4):575-602.

[36] Ruschena D, Mullen PE, Palmer S, Burgess P, Cordner SM, Drummer OH, et al., Choking deaths: the role of antipsychotic medication. *Br. J. Psychiatry J. Ment Sci.* nov 2003;183:446-50.

[37] Winkelman JW. Schizophrenia, obesity, and obstructive sleep apnea. *J. Clin. Psychiatry.* janv 2001;62(1):8-11.

[38] Filik R, Sipos A, Kehoe PG, Burns T, Cooper SJ, Stevens H, et al., The cardiovascular and respiratory health of people with schizophrenia. *Acta Psychiatr Scand.* avr 2006;113(4):298‑305.

[39] Chen Y-H, Lin H-C, Lin H-C. Poor clinical outcomes among pneumonia patients with schizophrenia. *Schizophr Bull.* sept 2011;37(5):1088‑94.

[40] Bushe CJ, Bradley AJ, Wildgust HJ, Hodgson RE. Schizophrenia and breast cancer incidence: a systematic review of clinical studies. *Schizophr Res.* oct 2009;114(1-3):6‑16.

[41] Grinshpoon A, Barchana M, Ponizovsky A, Lipshitz I, Nahon D, Tal O, et al., Cancer in schizophrenia: is the risk higher or lower? *Schizophr Res.* 1 mars 2005;73(2-3):333‑41.

[42] Carlsen K, Høybye MT, Dalton SO, Tjønneland A. Social inequality and incidence of and survival from breast cancer in a population-based study in Denmark, 1994-2003. *Eur. J. Cancer Oxf. Engl 1990.* sept 2008;44(14):1996‑2002.

[43] Hippisley-Cox J, Vinogradova Y, Coupland C, Parker C. Risk of malignancy in patients with schizophrenia or bipolar disorder: nested case-control study. *Arch. Gen. Psychiatry.* déc 2007;64(12):1368‑76.

[44] Dalton SO, Mellemkjaer L, Thomassen L, Mortensen PB, Johansen C. Risk for cancer in a cohort of patients hospitalized for schizophrenia in Denmark, 1969-1993. *Schizophr Res.* 15 juin 2005;75(2-3):315‑24.

[45] De Hert M, Cohen D, Bobes J, Cetkovich-Bakmas M, Leucht S, Ndetei DM, et al., Physical illness in patients with severe mental disorders. II. Barriers to care, monitoring and treatment guidelines, plus recommendations at the system and individual level. World Psychiatry *Off J. World Psychiatr Assoc WPA.* juin 2011;10(2):138‑51.

[46] Haddad PM, Sharma SG. Adverse effects of atypical antipsychotics: differential risk and clinical implications. *CNS Drugs.* 2007;21(11):911‑36.

[47] Flanagan RJ, Dunk L. Haematological toxicity of drugs used in psychiatry. *Hum. Psychopharmacol.* janv 2008;23 Suppl 1:27‑41.

[48] Dinwiddie SH, Shicker L, Newman T. Prevalence of hepatitis C among psychiatric patients in the public sector. *Am. J. Psychiatry.* janv 2003;160(1):172‑4.

[49] Schaefer M, Hinzpeter A, Mohmand A, Janssen G, Pich M, Schwaiger M, et al., Hepatitis C treatment in « difficult-to-treat » psychiatric patients with pegylated interferon-alpha and ribavirin: response and psychiatric side effects. *Hepatol. Baltim Md.* oct 2007;46(4):991‑8.

[50] Meade CS, Sikkema KJ. HIV risk behavior among adults with severe mental illness: a systematic review. *Clin. Psychol. Rev.* juin 2005;25(4):433‑57.

[51] Müller N, Wagner JK, Krause D, Weidinger E, Wildenauer A, Obermeier M, et al., Impaired monocyte activation in schizophrenia. *Psychiatry Res.* 15 août 2012;198(3):341‑6.

[52] Yovel G, Sirota P, Mazeh D, Shakhar G, Rosenne E, Ben-Eliyahu S. Higher natural killer cell activity in schizophrenic patients: the impact of serum factors, medication, and smoking. *Brain Behav. Immun.* sept 2000;14(3):153‑69.

[53] Drake RE, Mercer-McFadden C, Mueser KT, McHugo GJ, Bond GR. Review of integrated mental health and substance abuse treatment for patients with dual disorders. *Schizophr Bull.* 1998;24(4):589-608.

[54] Brennan PA, Mednick SA, Hodgins S. Major mental disorders and criminal violence in a Danish birth cohort. *Arch. Gen. Psychiatry.* mai 2000;57(5):494-500.

[55] Autié A, Montreuil M, Moulier V, Braha S, Wojakiewicz A, Januel D. [Pain and schizophrenia: myth and reality]. *L'Encéphale.* sept 2009;35(4):297-303.

[56] Malmo RB, Shagass C, Smith AA. Responsiveness in chronic schizophrenia. *J. Pers.* juin 1951;19(4):359-75.

[57] Singh MK, Giles LL, Nasrallah HA. Pain insensitivity in schizophrenia: trait or state marker? *J. Psychiatr Pract.* mars 2006;12(2):90-102.

[58] DE Hert M, Correll CU, Bobes J, Cetkovich-Bakmas M, Cohen D, Asai I, et al., Physical illness in patients with severe mental disorders. I. Prevalence, impact of medications and disparities in health care. *World Psychiatry Off J. World Psychiatr Assoc WPA.* févr 2011;10(1):52-77.

[59] Lenander-Lumikari M, Loimaranta V. Saliva and dental caries. *Adv. Dent. Res.* déc 2000;14:40-7.

[60] Petersen PE, Bourgeois D, Ogawa H, Estupinan-Day S, Ndiaye C. The global burden of oral diseases and risks to oral health. *Bull World Health Organ* [Internet]. sept 2005 [cité 24 janv 2015];83(9):661-9. Disponible sur: http://www.ncbi.nlm.nih.gov/pmc/articles/ PMC2626328/

[61] Shah VR, Jain P, Patel N. Oral health of psychiatric patients: A cross-sectional comparision study. *Dent Res. J.* [Internet]. 2012 [cité 12 janv 2015];9(2):209-14. Disponible sur: http://www.ncbi.nlm.nih.gov/ pmc/articles/PMC3353700/

[62] DeBaz C, Shamia H, Hahn J, Mithani S, Sadeghi G, Palomo L. Periodontitis impacts quality of life in postmenopausal women. *Climacteric J. Int. Menopause Soc.* 2 janv 2015;1-14.

[63] Ramon T, Grinshpoon A, Zusman SP, Weizman A. Oral health and treatment needs of institutionalized chronic psychiatric patients in Israel. *Eur. Psychiatry J. Assoc. Eur. Psychiatr.* mai 2003;18(3):101-5.

[64] Awartani F. Evaluation of the relationship between type 2 diabetes and periodontal disease. *Odonto-Stomatol. Trop Trop Dent J.* déc 2009;32(128):33-9.

[65] Simpson TC, Needleman I, Wild SH, Moles DR, Mills EJ. Treatment of periodontal disease for glycaemic control in people with diabetes. *Cochrane Database Syst. Rev.* 2010;(5):CD004714.

[66] Zelkha SA, Freilich RW, Amar S. Periodontal innate immune mechanisms relevant to atherosclerosis and obesity. *Periodontol. 2000.* oct 2010;54(1):207-21.

[67] Morita I, Okamoto Y, Yoshii S, Nakagaki H, Mizuno K, Sheiham A, et al., Five-year incidence of periodontal disease is related to body mass index. *J. Dent Res.* févr 2011;90(2):199-202.

[68] Romagna C, Dufour L, Troisgros O, Lorgis L, Richard C, Buffet P, et al., Periodontal disease: a new factor associated with the presence of multiple complex coronary lesions. *J. Clin. Periodontol.* janv 2012;39(1):38-44.

[69] Arnaiz A, Zumárraga M, Díez-Altuna I, Uriarte JJ, Moro J, Pérez-Ansorena MA. Oral health and the symptoms of schizophrenia. *Psychiatry Res.* 30 juin 2011;188(1):24-8.

[70] Chu K-Y, Yang N-P, Chou P, Chiu H-J, Chi L-Y. Comparison of oral health between inpatients with schizophrenia and disabled people or the general population. *J. Formos Med Assoc. Taiwan Yi Zhi.* avr 2012;111(4):214-9.

[71] Eltas A, Kartalcı S, Eltas SD, Dündar S, Uslu MO. An assessment of periodontal health in patients with schizophrenia and taking antipsychotic medication. *Int. J. Dent Hyg.* mai 2013;11(2):78-83.

[72] Nikfarjam M, Parvin N. Oral health status in three long term care units of schizophrenic patients in chaharmahal-bakhtiari province, iran. *Iran Red. Crescent Med. J.* avr 2013;15(4):371-2.

[73] Chu K-Y, Yang N-P, Chou P, Chi L-Y, Chiu H-J. Dental prosthetic treatment needs of inpatients with schizophrenia in Taiwan: a cross-sectional study. *BMC Oral Health.* 2013;13:8.

[74] Chu K-Y, Yang N-P, Chou P, Chi L-Y, Chiu H-J. The relationship between body mass index, the use of second-generation antipsychotics, and dental caries among hospitalized patients with schizophrenia. *Int. J. Psychiatry Med.* 2011;41(4):343-53.

[75] Chu K-Y, Yang N-P, Chou P, Chiu H-J, Chi L-Y. Factors associated with dental caries among institutionalized residents with schizophrenia in Taiwan: a cross-sectional study. *BMC Public Health.* 2010;10:482.

[76] Tani H, Uchida H, Suzuki T, Shibuya Y, Shimanuki H, Watanabe K, et al., Dental conditions in inpatients with schizophrenia: a large-scale multi-site survey. *BMC Oral Health.* 2012;12:32.

[77] Nielsen J, Munk-Jørgensen P, Skadhede S, Correll CU. Determinants of poor dental care in patients with schizophrenia: a historical, prospective database study. *J. Clin. Psychiatry.* févr 2011;72(2):140-3.

[78] McCreadie RG, Stevens H, Henderson J, Hall D, McCaul R, Filik R, et al., The dental health of people with schizophrenia. *Acta Psychiatr Scand.* oct 2004;110(4):306-10.

[79] Capdevielle D, Ritchie K, Villebrun D, Boulenger J-P. [Schizophrenic patients' length of stay: clinical factors of variability and consequences]. *L'Encéphale.* févr 2009;35(1):90-6.

[80] Janardhanan T, Cohen CI, Kim S, Rizvi BF. Dental care and associated factors among older adults with schizophrenia. *J. Am. Dent Assoc.* 1939. janv 2011;142(1):57-65.

[81] Szöke A, Trandafir A, Dupont M-E, Méary A, Schürhoff F, Leboyer M. Longitudinal studies of cognition in schizophrenia: meta-analysis. *Br. J. Psychiatry J Ment Sci.* avr 2008;192(4):248-57.

[82] Sartorius N. Stigmatized illnesses and health care. *Croat Med. J.* juin 2007;48(3):396-7.

[83] Mitchell BD. Clustering of schizophrenia with other comorbidities--what can we learn? *Schizophr Bull.* mars 2009;35(2):282-3.

[84] effehs.pdf [Internet]. [cité 24 janv 2015]. Disponible sur: http://homepage.hispeed.ch/Jerome_Favrod/effehs.pdf

[85] Ponizovsky AM, Zusman SP, Dekel D, Masarwa A-S, Ramon T, Natapov L, et al., Effect of implementing dental services in Israeli psychiatric hospitals on the oral and dental health of inpatients. *Psychiatr Serv. Wash DC.* juin 2009;60(6):799-803.

[86] Fratto G, Manzon L. Use of psychotropic drugs and associated dental diseases. *Int. J. Psychiatry Med.* 2014;48(3):185-97.

[87] Friedlander AH, Marder SR. The psychopathology, medical management and dental implications of schizophrenia. *J Am Dent Assoc* 1939. mai 2002;133(5):603-10; quiz 624-5.

[88] Gouzien C, Valiamé A, Misdrahi D. [Clozapine-induced parotitis: a case study]. *L'Encéphale.* févr 2014;40(1):81-5.

[89] Khokhar WA, Clifton A, Jones H, Tosh G. Oral health advice for people with serious mental illness. *Cochrane Database Syst. Rev.* 2011;(11):CD008802.

[90] Kisely S, Smith M, Lawrence D, Cox M, Campbell LA, Maaten S. Inequitable access for mentally ill patients to some medically necessary procedures. *CMAJ Can. Med. Assoc. J. J. Assoc. Medicale Can.* 13 mars 2007;176(6):779-84.

[91] Khokhar WA, Clifton A, Jones H, Tosh G. Oral health advice for people with serious mental illness. *Cochrane Database Syst Rev.* 2011;(11):CD008802.

[92] Staudte H, Kranz S, Völpel A, Schütze J, Sigusch BW. Comparison of nutrient intake between patients with periodontitis and healthy subjects. *Quintessence Int. Berl. Ger.* 1985. déc 2012;43(10):907-16.

[93] Druss BG, Bornemann TH. Improving health and health care for persons with serious mental illness: the window for US federal policy change. *JAMA.* 19 mai 2010;303(19):1972-3.

[94] Oral Health Care for People with Mental Health Problems_Guidelines and Recommendations - BSDH2000.pdf [Internet]. [cité 18 janv 2015]. Disponible sur: https://www.adelaide.edu.au/oral-health-promotion/resources/prof/htm_files/BSDH2000.pdf

In: Oral Health
Editor: Julia Renee Barnes
ISBN: 978-1-63482-832-1

Chapter VII

Oral Health and the Quality of Life for Romanian Orthodontic Patients

Irina Zetu, Sorana Rosu*, Liviu Zetu and Mihnea Iacob
"Grigore T. Popa" University of Medicine and Pharmacy, Iasi, Romania

Abstract

Objectives: *Psychosocial Impact of Dental Aesthetic Questionnaire* (PIDAQ) represents the only available tool for assessing the quality of life for the orthodontic patients. The research studied the relationships between the different aspects of orthodontic care planning, and validated the Romanian version of the PIDAQ questionnaire.

Material and methods: A transversal study was carried out on a sample of 1126 subjects, age ranging between 6 and 28 years old. The self-evaluation of the orthodontic esthetic perception was assessed with the PIDAQ index, and the orthodontic treatment need was measured with the IOTN index.

Results: Esthetic perception - 70% of the subjects are unsatisfied with the appearance of their dentition.

Orthodontic treatment need perception - All the subjects consider that they need orthodontic treatment.

Esthetic perception and orthodontic treatment need relationship - 40.16% of the subjects, which were unsatisfied with their dentition appearance, considered that they do not require an orthodontic treatment.

Esthetic perception and the esthetic component of IOTN correlation - Among the subjects, assessed as in need severe treatment, 80% were "Unsatisfied" or "Deeply unsatisfied" with their dentition.

Discussion: The scores of the different PIDAQ dimensions determined in our study, were comparable with those reported by other authors.

Conclusion: The PIDAQ questionnaire remains the only tool to assess the link between the dental-maxillary anomalies and the quality of life.

* Corresponding author: Sorana Rosu. E-mail: rosu_danut82@yahoo.com.

Our results demonstrate that the Romanian version of the PIDAQ questionnaire is a valid instrument in assessing the psychosocial impact of the dentition esthetics related to the malocclusion.

Introduction

Psychosocial Impact of Dental Aesthetic Questionnaire PIDAQ, developed in 2006 by Klages and co-workers, represents the only available tool designed specifically to assess malocclusions [1].

PIDAQ represents a validated indicator for assessing the quality of life in relation to the oral health, specific to the field of orthodontics. This self-administered questionnaire was assembled by the means of the preliminary studies by Klages and co-workers, in 2004 and 2005 [191], which were inspired by OQLQ (Orthognatic *Quality of Life Questionnaire*) or *Cunningham* and co-workers Questionnaire [2].

PIDAQ's main objective is to evaluate the psycho-social impact of the dental aesthetics. It may also be used to assess: the orthodontic treatment need, the orthodontic treatment results, the orthodontic treatment gains at psycho-social levels and also as a research tool for studies related to the oral health of the orthodontic patient.

Initially developed and tested on groups of young adults, these concepts seem to be equally useful for children and adolescents.

PIDAQ analyses four fundamental fields:

- Self-confidence;
- Social impact;
- Psychological impact;
- Aesthetic needs.

Each field comprises of a different number of items, six for "self-confidence," eight for "social impact," six for "psychological impact" and three for "aesthetic needs." PIDAQ includes in total 23 items that the patient must assess, using a Likert type scale in five steps: total disagree, disagree, no option, agree, total agree.

Our research had as primary objectives to assess the relationships between the different aspects of the orthodontic care forecasts (the psychometric properties of the questionnaire) and to validate the Romanian version of the PIDAQ questionnaire.

Material and Methods

A transversal study was conducted using a group of 1126 subjects.

The orthodontic aesthetic self-perception and the orthodontic treatment need of each subject were assessed with the help of Psycho-social Impact of Dental Aesthetic (PIDAQ).

The same questionnaire was used to record the potential impact of malocclusion on each subject quality of life.

We also evaluated each subject's need of orthodontic treatment by means of the Index of Orthodontic treatment Need - IOTN.

The study group consisted of 1126 subjects, some of which had already undergone orthodontic treatment. Most subjects were first evaluated by an orthodontics specialist.

The subjects' ages ranged from 6 to 28 years old. All study participants were volunteers, who had received exhaustive information about the study and signed an informed consent form.

Data gathering: Four types of data were gathered from all the study group subjects:

- Social-demographics (age, sex)
- Orthodontic aesthetics perception
- Orthodontic treatment need
- Malocclusion- quality of life relationship

Table I presents the used variables and their nature. The qualitative variables (sex, the orthodontic treatment need described by IOTN – AC and DHC) were presented as absolute actual value and as percentage. The importance of the potential association, between these variables, was evaluated using the χ^2 (Khi-2) test.

The scores of the different PIDAQ's questionnaire parameters presented a normal distribution, as they were evaluated with the Kolmogorov-Smirnov test. They were described as mean values and ecart-types. The independent samples t test was used to assess the association between the dependent and independent variables (sex, aesthetic perception, orthodontic treatments need self-perception, and orthodontic treatment needs are indicated by IOTN).

The other quantitative variables (the personal perception of the orthodontic aesthetics, the subjective orthodontic treatment need or request) were regarded as quantitative systematized variables. They were described by absolute value and percentage. Their association was tested by a Spearman correlation.

Table 1. The list of the studied variables

Parameter	Variable	Variables Nature	Measure Unit
Orthodontic treatment need	IOTN AC	Qualitative binary	Without
	IOTN DHC		
Social – Demographic Variable	Sex	Qualitative binary	Without
	Age	Quantitative continue	Years
Life quality (PIDAQ)	Self confidence	Quantitative continue	Without
	Social Impact		
	Psychological Impact		
	Aesthetic needs		
Aesthetic perception		Quantitative continue	Without
Orthodontic treatment need self-perception		Quantitative continue	Without

The Personal Perception of Orthodontic Aesthetics

The perception, which the patient had about his/hers dental arches alignment (the orthodontic aesthetic), was evaluated by the question –"Are you satisfied with the alignment of your teeth"

- "unsatisfied"
- "a bit satisfied"
- "moderately satisfied"
- "satisfied"
- "very satisfied"

The Subjective Perception of the Orthodontic Treatment Need

Even if some of the patients were already investigated for orthodontic issues, we considered it important to also test the subjective perception of an orthodontic treatment need, by the question – "Do you believe that you need orthodontic treatment?"
The possible choices were:

"No, not at all"
- "No, I don't think so"
- "I believe I do"
- "Yes, I am sure"

We found the patient was not always the one requesting the appointment with the orthodontist. This was the case for the small children, but also for some adults, who had been pressured by their entourage.

The Normative Evaluation of the Orthodontic Treatment Need

The normative evaluation of the orthodontic treatment needed was evaluated with the IOTN index. This index comprises an aesthetic component, which involves a photographic ten steps scale, and a dental health scale, which assesses five levels of malocclusion, missing teeth, over jet, overbite and open bite.

In the first stage the orthodontic aesthetics was evaluated by the investigator, using the photographic scale, where the photo number 1 was the most attractive occlusion, and photo number ten, the least attractive. The doctor evaluated the occlusion, with no treatment prognosis involved, discarding the teeth colorations, the cavities, gingival problems, the evaluation being only aesthetic.

The dental health component of the IOTN was registered with a special ruler.

PIDAQ Questionnaire Validation

In order to validate the PIDAQ questionnaire, we used the version that included 23 elements, grouped in four domains: aesthetic aspect, psychological impact, social impact, and self-confidence.

The PIDAQ questionnaire was translated from English into Romanian by two translators, who worked separately and then together for the final version. This final version was again translated into English.

Two orthodontists and one dentist, who were previously calibrated using the PIDAQ, conducted the clinical examinations and the filling out of the questionnaires.

PIDAQ Validation Study Group

In order to validate the Romanian version of the PIDAQ, we selected a study group of 152 dental medicine students, from the School of Dental Medicine "Grigore T. Popa" University, Iasi. The conclusion was that the Romanian version of the questionnaire was correctly translated and adapted.

Evaluation of the Validity and Viability of PIDAQ Romanian Version

The exclusion criteria were: subjects with cavities or traumas on the frontal teeth, dental hypoplasia, fluoride-induced lesions, and subjects undergoing orthodontic treatment.

IOTN Evaluation

The aesthetic component of the IOTN was utilized, the clinical examination being conducted by two orthodontists and one dentist, previously calibrated (Kappa >0.85).

The results were separated into three groups: score 1-4, 5-7 and 8-10.

Statistical Analysis

We used the SPSS 20.0 for Windows for the statistical analysis. The results were obtained by descriptive analysis (mean and standard deviation for each variable). Internal consistency, measured with Cronbach´s alpha test, was also calculated.

The PIDAQ viability was calculated by measuring the interclass correlation coefficient. The validity was determined by comparing the IOTN-AC scores with the scores for each subscale and the whole PIDAQ test. The mean values were compared with the ANOVA test.

Ethical Consideration

The study was approved by the Ethics Commission of the "Grigore T. Popa" University, Iasi.

Results

The internal consistency index of the questionnaire, determined by the Cronbach´s alpha test was 0.926, while the minimal standard value is 0.912, which signifies that the Romanian version of the PIDAQ questionnaire presented a good degree of viability (Table 2).

The values obtained for the questionnaire's question ranged between 0.39 and 0.69. The mean viability for the under scales was 0.855 for confidence, 0.932 for social impact, 0.919 psychological impact and 0.880 aesthetic aspect. The correlation coefficient was >0.397.

PIDAQ Questionnaire Validity

The test Kaiser-Meyer-Olkin valued 0.929, and Bartlett´s test scored 6271.919 (p = 0.00) (Table 3). The common factor 1 contains the question from the social impact section (questions 7-14) (eigenvalue = 0.148) and sustains 0.65% of the variables. The common factor 2 contains the question from the confidence section (questions 1-6 (eigenvalue = 3.5)) and sustains 15.5% of the variables.

The common factor 3 contains the question from the psychosocial impact section (questions 15-20) (eigenvalue = 0.5) and sustains 0.12% of the variables. The common factor 4, questions 21-23, the aesthetic aspect section (eigenvalue = 0.015) explains 0.066% of the variant.

Reproducibility

The reproducibility of the PIDAQ was assessed by determining the degree of interclass correlation index, which scored 0.926, ranging between 0.908 and 0.942 for the four scales below (Table 5).

Table 2. The viability degree analysis

Cronbach's Alpha	Cronbach's Alpha Based on Standardized Items	N of Items
.926	.912	22

Table 3. KMO and Bartlett's Test

Kaiser-Meyer-Olkin Measure of Sampling Adequacy.		.929
Bartlett's Test of Sphericity	Approx. Chi-Square	6271.919
	df	253
	Sig.	.000

Table 4. Presents the results for each separate question

Table VII.4 Rotated Component Matrix[a]				
	Component			
	1	2	3	4
. I am proud of my teeth.			.872	
I like to show my teeth when I smile.			.873	
I am pleased when I see my teeth in the mirror.			.903	
My teeth are attractive to others.			.896	
. I am satisfied with the appearance of my teeth.			.789	
. I find my tooth position to be very nice			.801	
. I hold myself back when I smile so my teeth don't show so much.	.913			
. If I don't know people well I am sometimes concerned what they might think about my teeth.	.948			
I'm afraid other people could make offensive remarks about my teeth.	.952			
. I am somewhat inhibited in social contacts because of my teeth.	.933			
. I sometimes catch myself holding my hand in front of my mouth to hide my teeth.	.934			
Sometimes I think people are staring at my teeth.	.905			
Remarks about my teeth irritate me even when they are meant jokingly.	.956			
I sometimes worry about what members of the opposite sex think about my teeth.	.916			
I envy the nice teeth of other people.		.891		
. I am somewhat distressed when I see other people's teeth.		.937		
. Sometimes I am somewhat unhappy about the appearance of my teeth.		.919		
I think most people I know have nicer teeth than I do.		.935		
. I feel bad when I think about what my teeth look like.		.936		
. I wish my teeth looked better		.894		
. I envy the nice teeth of other people.				.885
. I am somewhat distressed when I see other people's teeth.				.875
. Sometimes I am somewhat unhappy about the appearance of my teeth.				.886
Extraction Method: Principal Component Analysis. Rotation Method: Varimax with Kaiser Normalization.[a]				

[a]Rotation converged in 5 iterations.

Results and Discussions

The scores for the different PIDAQ domains are indicated in Table 6. As absolute value, the social impact presented the highest score (13.72), but it also includes the highest items number.

In order to avoid the item number influence, the rate between the scores mean and the maximum possible score was calculated. The aesthetic needs present the biggest impact, with a rate of 0.47. For this type of evaluation, confidence presents the lowest impact. The intraclass coefficient ranges from 0.72 for "Social Impact" to 0.90 for "Aesthetic needs" (Table 7).

Table 5. Intraclass Correlation Coefficient

	Intraclass Correlation[b]	95% Confidence Interval		F Test with True Value 0			
		Lower Bound	Upper Bound	Value	df1	df2	Sig
Single Measures	.362[a]	.308	.424	13.462	151	3171	0.000
Average Measures	.926[c]	.908	.942	13.462	151	3171	0.000

For all the statistic tests the significance limit was set at $p \leq 0.05$.

Table 6. Scores and Viability (internal coherence and PIDAQ questionnaire reproducibility)

Dimensions (items number)	Mean ± Ecart Type	Maximum possible score	Mean / maxim score
Confidence (6)	6.84±6.1	30	0.23
Social Impact(8)	13.72±13.33	40	0.34
Psychological Impact (6)	12.21±10.42	30	0.40
Aesthetic need (3)	7.07±4.36	15	0.47

The internal coherence of the items for each domain varies from 0.67 for "Aesthetic needs" to 0.87 for "Social Impact."

Table 7. PIDAQ's domains viability

Dimensions (Items number)	Viability	
	Internal coherence	Reproducibility
	Coefficient α Cronbach	Intra-class correlation coefficient
Confidence (6)	0.71	0.73
Social Impact(8)	0.87	0.72
Psychological Impact (6)	0.79	0.85
Aesthetic perception (3)	0.67	0.90

The association between the different domains of the PIDAQ, the aesthetic perception, and the perceived need was tested by a Spearman correlation.

Table 7 shows the correlation matrix between these different variables. The patient perception of their dental alignment is significantly correlated with three domains of the PIDAQ (Social Impact, Psychological Impact and Aesthetic needs). On the other hand, the perceived need is not significantly correlated with any of the PIDAQ needs.

Study Results

Social - Demographic Characteristics

Table 9 presents the social-demographic distribution. Females represent 50.03% of the included subjects; most females in the study group were older than the boys, but there was no statistically significant difference between the males and females mean ages (p = 0,25). The males mean age was also inferior to the study groups mean age.

Aesthetic Perception

Table 10 presents the distribution of the degree of subject satisfaction regarding their occlusion. It seems that almost 70% are, at different rates, unsatisfied with the orthodontic aesthetics of their occlusion.

Table 8. Spearman correlation matrix

	Aesthetic perception rho (p)	Perceived need rho (p)
Confidence (6)	0.20 (0.20)	-0.05 (0.74)
Social Impact (8)	-0.35* (0.02)	0.29 (0.16)
Psychological Impact (6)	-0.34* (0.02)	0.20 (0.19)
Aesthetic perception (3)	-0.43* (0.004)	0.22 (0.16)

Table 9. Social- demographic variables distribution

Age		Test t. p Value
Sex	Male (n = 559)	0.25
	Female (n = 567)	
	Total (n = 1126)	

Table 10. Perceived orthodontic aesthetics - Scores distribution

	Subjects perception of their occlusion %					Test χ2 Value p
M (n = 559)	Very unsatisfied	Unsatisfied	Moderately satisfied	Satisfied	Very satisfied	0.25
	224 (40.07)	126 (22.54)	17 (3.04)	77 (13.77)	117 (20.58)	
F (n = 567)	217 (38.27)	182 (32.08)	38 (6.7)	17 (2.99)	113 (19.96)	
Total (n = 1126)	441 (41)	308 (27.35)	55 (4.88)	94 (8.34)	230 (20.42)	

Table 11. Scores for perceived treatment need

	Orthodontic treatment need perception n%					Test χ2 Value p
M (n = 559)	No. Not at all	No. I don't think so	No option	Yes. I think so	Yes. I am sure of it	0.68
	20 (3.67)	55 (9.83)	125 (22.36)	134 (23.97)	225 (40.17)	
F (n = 567)	53 (9.34)	76 (13.40)	60 (10.58)	151 (26.63)	227 (40.05)	
Total (n = 1126)	73 (6.48)	131 (11.63)	185 (16.42)	285 (25.31)	452 (40.16)	

This dissatisfaction interests 70.35% of the females, and 62.61% of the males. The $\chi 2$ test presents no significant difference ($p = 0.25$).

Orthodontic Treatment Needs Perception or the Perceived or Requested Treatment Need

All the subjects included into this study presume or are sure that their occlusion requires orthodontic treatment. Of these, 45% are certain that they need treatment (Table 11). Belonging to a specific group does not influence the perceived orthodontic treatment need ($p = 0.68$).

Aesthetic Perception and Requested Need Relationship

Interestingly, 40.16% of the subjects who are very unsatisfied with their teeth alignment are not certain that an orthodontic treatment is necessary (Figure 1).

The subjects that are very satisfied or moderately satisfied with their teeth alignment declared that they require orthodontic treatment (Figure 1). Aesthetic perception analysis shows that it does not significantly influence the treatment request or the perceived need ($p = 0.30$).

Aesthetic Perception and the Normative Treatment Need (IOTN-AC) Relation

Eighty percent of the subjects, whose evaluation of the aesthetic component of the IOTN classified as a severe need of treatment, are very unsatisfied or unsatisfied with their occlusions. The rest of the subjects are moderately satisfied with their dental arch alignment. Almost half of the subjects who do not require orthodontic treatment, as evaluated by the IOTN (AC), declared that they are very satisfied with their dental alignment (Figure 2).

The association between the orthodontic aesthetic perception and the normative treatment need (IOTN) is not significant.

Discussion

Different aspects of the orthodontic treatment need forecast, were analysed – aesthetics, perceived or required need, normative need and the quality of life.

Limitations

One of the limitations of this study is related to the fact that many subjects were seeking orthodontic treatment. In fact, some of them had already started an orthodontic treatment.

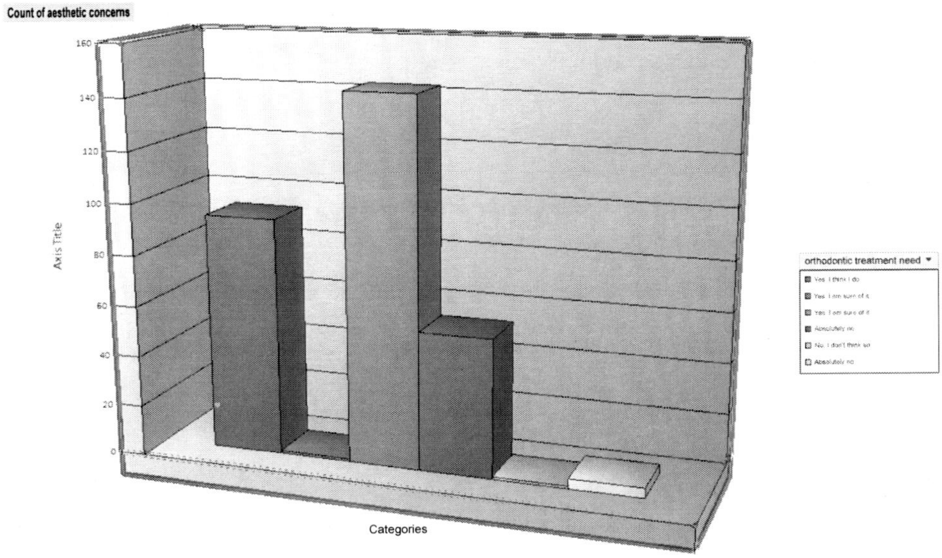

Figure 1. Aesthetic perception and requested need relationship.

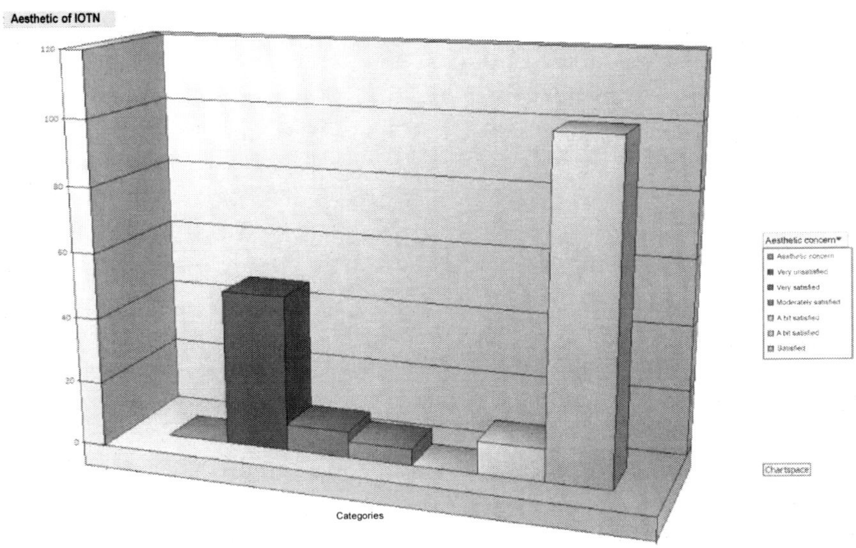

Figure 2. Aesthetic perceptions and the normative treatment need (IOTN-AC) relation.

It might be presumed that the motivation of these patients is strong. In fact, many times, the beneficiary of the orthodontic treatment is not the person who initiated the appointment. For children and adolescents, the parents are the ones who seek the best facial and dental appearance for their offspring [3, 4]. In adult patients, the pressure can often come from the immediate entourage (husband, brother), orthodontic treatment not being the patients chief concern. Another limitation is related to the fact that the studied population, comprised mainly of adolescent and adult patients, some of whom had already been engaged in orthodontic treatment, and the gathered data describe a situation that they already encountered. A positive fact is that only a small number of the subjects were in this situation, and, also, recent research has reported that individuals keep intact memories involving their morphological anomalies for a long period of time [5]. It also should be noted that the male and female subjects were almost equally distributed, reflecting the percentages encountered for the orthodontic adult patients.

Aesthetics, Perceived Need and Normative Need

The evaluation by the patients of the degree of satisfaction related to their dental alignment (The orthodontic aesthetics) shows that 80% are unsatisfied. The question "Do you think that you need an orthodontic treatment" received 100% affirmative answers.

The perceived need involves all the patients, but 20% of them are not unsatisfied with their dental alignment. If we consider that the orthodontic aesthetics remains the principal motive for seeking treatment [6], we might ask ourselves what was the motivation for this particular group of patients. It might be the situation of patients referred by the dentist, with important malocclusions (lateral cross bite, posterior tooth agenesis), but who do not necessarily present aesthetic issues. The scores for the different PIDAQ domains calculated in our study are comparable with those reported in the orthodontic literature [7, 8]. The traditional orthodontic diagnosis avoids starting clinically unjustified treatments. An analysis of the relationship between the perceived and the normative need shows that differences are present. The perceived need, as evaluated by this study, is greater than the normative need. These differences were reported in large samples of population studies [9, 10, 11].

Conclusion

- until now, the PIDAQ questionnaire remains the only specific instrument for orthodontics, which relates malocclusion and the quality of life
- the result analysis demonstrates that PIDAQ has a very good psychometrical quality, and a good viability
- the internal coherence is very good, and the reproducibility is almost perfect, with an intra-class coefficient, which ranges from 0.72 for social-impact to 0.90 for aesthetic perception
- the scores of the different PIDAQ in our research domains are comparable to the other three studies, which used PIDAQ
- the Romanian version of the PIDAQ represents a useful tool for evaluation of the psycho-social impact of the dental aesthetic in relation with the malocclusion, in order to appreciate the quality of life of the Romanian orthodontic patients.

References

[1] Cunningham, S. J., Hunt, N. P. Are pre-treatment psychological characteristics influenced by pre-surgical orthodontics? *Eur. J. Orthod.* 2001;23:751–758.

[2] Birkeland, K., Bøe, O. E., Wisth, P. J. Relationship between occlusion and satisfaction with dental appearance in orthodontically treated and untreated groups. A longitudinal study. *Eur. J. Orthod.* 2000;22:509–518.

[3] World Health Organization (WHO). *Oral Health Surveys: Basic Methods.* 4th ed. Geneva: WHO; 1997.26.

[4] Jenny, J., Cons, N. C. *Guidelines for Using the DAI: A Supplement to DAI—The Dental Aesthetic Index.* Iowa City, Iowa: College of Dentistry, University of Iowa; 1988.

[5] Oliveira, B. H., Nadanovsky, P. Psychometric properties of the Brazilian version of the Oral Health Impact Profile-short form. *Community Dent. Oral Epidemiol.* 2005; 33: 307–314.

[6] Klages, U., Claus, N., Wehrbein, H., Zentner, A. Development of a questionnaire for assessment of the psychosocial impact of dental aesthetics in young adults. *Eur. J. Orthod.* 2006;28:103–111.

[7] O'Brien, C. O., Benson, P. E., Marshman, Z. Evaluation of a quality of life measure for children with malocclusion. *J. Orthod.* 2007; 34:185–193.

[8] Birkeland, K., Bøe, O. E., Wisth, P. J. Orthodontic concern among 11-year-old children, and their parents compared with orthodontic treatment need assessed by Index of Orthodontic Treatment Need. *Am. J. Orthod. Dentofacial. Orthop.* 1996; 110:197–205.

[9] Slade, G. D., Dewey, M. E., Newton, T., Brodie, P., Kiemle, G. Development and preliminary validation of the Body Satisfaction Scale (BSS). *Psychol. Health.* 1990;3: 213–220.

[10] Mandall, N. A., McCord, J. F., Blinkhorn, A. S., Worthington, H. V., O'Brien, K. D. Perceived aesthetic impact of malocclusion and oral self-perceptions in 14- to 15-year-old Asian and Caucasian children in greater Manchester. *Eur. J. Orthod.* 1999; 21:175–183.

[11] Al-Sarheed, M., Bedi, R., Hunt, N. P. Orthodontic treatment need and self-perception of 11- to 16-year-old Saudi Arabian children with a sensory impairment attending special schools. *J. Orthod.* 2003; 30:39–44.

Index

D

E

F

G

H

I

J

L

M

N

O

P

Q

R

S

T

U

V

W

X

Y

Z